Praise for *Upside*

"[Rendon's] book is designed to inspire and p
more fulfilled recovery. . . . The by no means ir
it contains scientifically grounded recommend
personal testimony about how it feels when you

—*Psychology Today*

"[*Upside*] tells the stories of nineteen people who survived combat, accidents, personal attacks, or disease, and who went on to remake their lives, find new narratives to propel them, and emerge stronger than before."

—*The Washington Post*

"It's deeply reassuring to know that no matter what one may go through in life, healing and growth—even luminous transformation—are still possible."

—*Spirituality & Health Magazine*

"An inspiring, empowering, and well-researched book."

—*Psych Central*

"Humorous, compassionate, friendly, and empathetic. . . . Rendon offers not just a spoonful of medicine, but also a furtherance of works by Frankl, Abraham Maslow, and his new, revitalized acquaintances."

—*Kirkus Reviews*

"None of us wants it, but severe stress may not be as bad as we think. *Upside* provides authentic hope, grounded in science and enlivened by real-life stories, that it is possible to emerge from a traumatic experience not diminished, but somehow enlarged by it. This book offers scientific evidence, personal understanding, and practical tools to transform trauma into an occasion for growth."

—Henry Emmons, MD, author of *The Chemistry of Joy*

"*Upside* is a true gift to the field of trauma recovery. The message can no longer be ignored. Post-traumatic growth is not only possible; it's our birthright."

—Linda Graham, MFT, author of *Bouncing Back:
Rewiring Your Brain for Maximum Resilience and Well-Being*

The New Science
of
Post-Traumatic Growth

UPSIDE

JIM RENDON

Touchstone

New York   London   Toronto   Sydney   New Delhi

Touchstone
An Imprint of Simon & Schuster, Inc.
1230 Avenue of the Americas
New York, NY 10020

First Touchstone paperback edition August 2016

TOUCHSTONE and colophon are registered trademarks of Simon & Schuster, Inc.

For information about special discounts for bulk purchases, please contact Simon & Schuster Special Sales at 1-866-506-1949 or business@simonandschuster.com.

The Simon & Schuster Speakers Bureau can bring authors to your live event. For more information or to book an event, contact the Simon & Schuster Speakers Bureau at 1-866-248-3049 or visit our website at www.simonspeakers.com.

Interior design by Akasha Archer

Manufactured in the United States of America

10 9 8 7 6 5 4 3 2 1

The Library of Congress has cataloged the hardcover edition as follows:

Rendon, Jim.
  The new science of post-traumatic growth / Jim Rendon.
    pages cm
  ISBN 978-1-4767-6163-3 (hardcover)—ISBN 978-1-4767-6164-0 (ebook) 1. Psychic trauma. 2. Post-traumatic stress disorder. 3. Life change events—Psychological aspects. I. Title.
  BF175.5.P75R46 2015
  155.9'042—dc23
                                                                    2015002864

ISBN 978-1-4767-6163-3
ISBN 978-1-4767-6165-7 (pbk)
ISBN 978-1-4767-6164-0 (ebook)

For my parents, Michael and Joyce Rendon

CONTENTS

PART THREE
Cultivating Growth

INTRODUCTION

My father, Michael Rendon, is a Holocaust survivor. So the question of how trauma changes people, how it shapes their lives and their sense of self, has always been part of my life.

He was just a teenager when German soldiers took him from his home in Poland and sent him to a concentration camp. He survived a winter death march from Poland to the Buchenwald concentration camp in Germany. From there he was moved to a smaller camp called Mittelbau-Dora. Even among concentration camps, this place was notorious. The Nazis forced prisoners to hollow out mines under the Harz Mountains, creating two parallel tunnels; each was 40 feet wide, 28 feet high, and nearly a mile long. Dozens of chambers ran between them. This complex became a vast subterranean factory that was impregnable to Allied bombs. In the belly of this mountain, prisoners built the VI and VII rockets that bombarded London. And while they worked, they risked their lives to sabotage those very rockets. They faked welds, left out parts, loosened screws. After rockets started malfunctioning, the guards' brutality increased—people were beaten to death, shot, or hung above the factory floor for the slightest infraction. The death rate at Dora was among the highest of any concentration camp.

In the mid-1990s, I visited Dora with my father. On a damp fall morning, as we walked around the former camp together, he explained the daily roll call that could go on for hours, showed me the tracks of the train that hauled parts and material into the rocket factory, even described as best he could what he saw every day inside the former mine. "Nobody could believe what was going on inside that tunnel. Inside was like hell. I don't think hell was like this," he told me. "People were falling like flies. There was no air. The dampness." We walked until we came to a rise near the tunnel entrances. I walked up to the chain link fence and craned my neck to get a better view—I wanted to see this place, get as close to it, to his experience, as I could. But here he held back. As he stared past the fence and into the shadows of the sealed tunnel entrances below, he became uncharacteristically quiet. He stood incredibly still for a moment and then slowly turned away.

My father talked about the war often. When I was young he told me fantastic adventure stories about the war and even comic stories that poked fun at the lazy, stupid guards. It wasn't until I was a teenager that he told me more about the horrors of his experience and how he escaped Dora.

Near the end of the war, as bombs from Allied planes fell around them, and guards and prisoners took cover, my father and a friend ran from Dora. The guards shot at them as they fled and he was wounded. He and his friend hid in the woods for two weeks, surviving on what they could scavenge or steal and trying to work their way to the American front. Over time, his wound became infected. He realized that if he was going to survive he needed medical attention. He stole the uniform from a dead SS officer and, wearing it, walked into an SS field hospital. At the end of the war the hospital was in chaos and no one asked too many questions. Medics cleaned his wound and bandaged him. He took a nap in one of the beds. When he woke up he saw a picture of Hitler hanging on the opposite wall. He got up, snuck out the door, and started running again.

When he finally came across American troops—soldiers in the 104th Infantry Division—they saw his SS uniform and thought he was a Nazi. Luckily one of the soldiers spoke Polish and my father explained that he had escaped from a concentration camp. Two days later the soldiers left him with the army's 20th Field Hospital, where he received a blood transfusion and care for his wound. He ate and regained his health. He is lucky that he escaped from Dora when he did. The Nazis killed nearly all of Dora's remaining prisoners in the waning days of the war.

My father told me that after he came to America, he joined the merchant marines so that he could divorce himself from the world. He wanted to simply sit on a ship in the middle of the ocean and just be left alone in a place where no one knew who he was, what he had survived, or what he had lost—his father, brother, stepmother, aunts, uncles, cousins, grandparents. Of his extended family of more than one hundred, only a few cousins survived the war.

Growing up, I often wondered how I would act in his place. What if an invading army rolled down my quiet New Jersey street and captured me? What would I do if I survived a concentration camp? Wouldn't I just crumble completely? I still don't know that I would have the strength to put one foot in front of the other and face the rest of my life. I marvel that my father has done that.

More recently, as young men and women began returning from Iraq and Afghanistan with post-traumatic stress disorder in increasing numbers, I began to wonder again about trauma and what it means to survive. What does a life-shattering trauma do to you? How does it change you? Can one ever bounce back from an experience like this? In the context of trauma does the phrase *bounce back* even mean anything? What I found amazed me, and gave me hope.

Most people have two opposing ideas about what it means to survive trauma. The first, and perhaps the most prevalent in our culture today, is that the event warps you, leaves you damaged and broken. It's the post-traumatic stress disorder so deeply associated with Vietnam War veterans and depicted in films like *The Deer Hunter*.

Following a traumatic event, most people experience a range of problems. They have nightmares and trouble sleeping. They are plagued by images of the traumatic event—reliving it over and over. They are on high alert, stuck in the thick of the brain's fear response. Many become anxious or depressed. The vast majority of people experience some of these post-traumatic stress symptoms, but they fade over time. Only a small percentage of people actually develop full-blown PTSD. A number of treatments have been developed for PTSD, but it remains a terrible and hard-to-treat condition, one that can take many years of therapy and medication to manage, one that can completely derail a life if left unattended.

Until recently, that was it. The whole discussion of the human response to trauma ended there: return to normal or suffer in the depths of PTSD. Therapy, medication, and psychological research have all been geared to helping people overcome this sometimes devastating post-trauma response with the goal of returning to normalcy.

But over the last few decades a small but growing group of researchers has found that trauma is more complex than that. A traumatic event, it turns out, is not simply a hardship to be overcome.

Instead, it is transformative. The trauma becomes a dividing line in survivors' lives. They are different after the event. Sometimes that change is negative—the post-traumatic stress symptoms that have received so much attention. But the changes don't end there. Trauma survivors are often pushed by a brush with their own mortality, by the depth of their hardship or even the suffering of others, to find more meaningful and fulfilling ways of understanding who they are and how they want to live. They struggle, but they also change for the better.

In a way it shouldn't be surprising that trauma can spark positive changes. Stories of people who rise from traumatic experience changed for the better can be found in cultures around the world. From our oldest heroic myths to the stories of the lives of sacred religious figures to superheroes in blockbuster movies like *Batman*, who watched as his parents were murdered and dedicated his life to battling crime, we learn over and over that traumatic events have the power to transform us into better people and make our lives more meaningful.

While descriptions of this phenomenon go back thousands of years, it was largely ignored by psychology. It was only in the 1980s that a handful of researchers began examining these beneficial changes. And what they found is startling. In study after study, research shows that about half or more of trauma survivors report positive changes as a result of their experience. Sometimes these are small changes—they feel that life has more meaning, that they are closer to their loved ones. For some the changes are life-altering, sending people on career and life paths they never would have considered before, transforming who they are and how they view the world. Every time I talk to one of these people in my reporting—someone who has totally altered his life, his sense of self, someone who says he is thankful for what most of us would consider a terrible tragedy—I am thrilled and amazed. What an exceptional person, I think. And then I remember all of the others who have told me similar stories. This kind of miraculous transformation, it turns out, is hardly unusual. The potential for such inspiring change lives inside most people.

My father was so young—just fourteen when the Germans invaded Poland—that his experiences during the war surely shaped him in profound ways. Like many of those I've met in the course of working on this book, he has never slept well. Since I was little he was always up at 5 a.m., weekday and weekend. His anxiety can be overwhelming. I joke with him that the Nazis won't shoot him if we are late for a dinner reservation. He usually looks at me like he's not so sure and goes to wait in the car. It's not long before the engine is running and he's laying on the horn.

Yet, at the same time, he has always had a remarkable sense of humor—he still tells those funny tales about life in the camps. He maintains close friendships. He has an outsize compassion for animals (stray dogs, cats, and injured birds were a fixture of my childhood home). When we visited Birkenau, the part of Auschwitz where he was unloaded from a boxcar as a terrified teenager all those years ago, he marveled at the sound of birds in nearby trees. He told me that when he was there during the war, he never heard a single bird.

I have never had the sense that he is bitter, but rather that he is accepting, coping, a survivor in the truest sense. When I asked my father if he thought that he had grown as a result of his experiences in the Holocaust, he said without missing a beat that he hadn't gone through anything like what today's soldiers experience in combat. I actually had to remind him that the Holocaust, though nearly seventy years behind him, was unquestionably horrific. But in his answer to my question about growth—the idea that the experience of others must be worse—is some clue to his point of view. He doesn't view his own situation as particularly terrible but rather empathizes with the traumatic experiences of others. He is quick to acknowledge the suffering of others. He has incredible inner strength. He, like so many who lost everything in the war, left his home country to start a new life here and succeeded. He told me that when he was in the merchant marines, he was on a ship moving seven thousand tons of explosives and munitions from Seattle to Korea for the war there. Many of his fellow sailors were jittery about spending ten days on a ship full of explosives. My father helped to calm them down. It's not that he wasn't afraid, but that he'd already been through so much worse. Sitting on a boat full of explosives where he had shelter, three meals a day, and air-conditioning, well, that was pretty good. His perspective was different from that of the sailors around him. All that he lived through, all that he survived, all that he lost, left him changed and some of those changes have been truly positive.

I hope that this book will help others suffering through the aftermath of a traumatic experience and will provide them with some of the tools they need to create a more positive future for themselves, perhaps even to transform their lives in ways they had never thought possible. And I hope to paint a more rounded picture of the aftermath of trauma—one with pain and suffering, to be sure, but one also filled with hope and opportunity for change.

PART ONE

Why Terrible Experiences Can Also Be Good for You

The Science Behind Trauma and Positive Change

CHAPTER 1

Reversing Psychology

How Two Researchers Discovered the
Transformative Power of Trauma

On a spring morning in 2009, Luther Delp sat on his pearl-white 1600 Kawasaki Vulcan motorcycle at a stoplight in Jacksonville, Florida. He loved that bike. Delp, who was fifty-nine years old at the time, had just put a thousand-dollar LED light system on the motorcycle so it could flash a multicolored glow on the road as he barreled down the highway. Even the wheels lit up. That spring morning he was on his way to Daytona Bike Week to buy a motorcycle for his wife, Debbie.

As Delp idled at the stoplight, a woman sped down the road in her car. She hadn't noticed the line of cars waiting for the light in front of her. And she never saw the motorcycle at the end of that line. She hit Delp at full speed. He was launched over three cars and landed on the fourth one with such force that he broke his back, multiple ribs, and his hips. He punctured his lung, and broke several teeth and his nose. His injuries were so catastrophic that he died right there at the intersection. Paramedics managed to revive him and then rushed him to the hospital. There he flatlined again and was revived once more. Doctors gave him twelve pints of blood. It poured through him.

Delp's blood pressure was so low that he couldn't take any painkillers for a torturous week while his doctors waited until he was strong enough to undergo surgery. The pain was overwhelming. "I was in so much pain. I told God, 'If this is all it is, please take me now,' " he says.

Butch and Cindy Davis were among the close friends who gathered in the waiting room with Delp's wife, Debbie. "We didn't think he was going to make it," says Davis. "We stayed in the hospital and held a vigil."

Davis and her husband met the Delps at a square dance thirty years before the accident. The couples quickly became close friends, vacationing together in their motorhomes. The Delps would stay up until two or three in the morning talking about their lives and planning new trips. They had plenty of time for whatever pursuit they could dream up. Delp had worked as a welder for twenty-seven years. He invested in real estate and retired in his forties. Now he and his wife were living comfortably off their investments. "All I did was play," says Delp. "I had a lot of time to go jet-skiing, ride motorcycles, go four-wheeling. We used to go dancing three or four nights a week. We camped and traveled all over the U.S." In the summers they went scalloping and waterskiing with Davis and her husband. They took cruises together with their children and grandchildren. Delp's parents had died when they were young and so he felt like he needed to experience as much as he could while he had the chance, says Cindy Davis. "We called him Lying Luther because you never knew what he was going to say next; he was a big kidder," she says.

Delp had been so active, so physical—always the first to slide under the camper to fix something—that Cindy couldn't imagine how he could live after such a catastrophic accident. "After such a trauma to his body, I didn't think that he wanted to pull through it," she says.

But Delp did survive. In the beginning he couldn't even sit up on his own. He lost movement and feeling in his legs and had little control over his torso. He developed bedsores. One on his backside grew so large and deep that Debbie could just about see through to the bone. She tried to keep things positive. "When I'd clean it and drain it, he'd ask, 'How does it look? Does it look any better?' and I'd tell him, 'Yeah, a little bit. A little bit,'" she says. "I didn't want to discourage him. If he saw it, he would have completely given up on life. I really believe that and so I didn't tell him."

Delp developed repeated infections. "Sometimes his fever would be so bad that he'd be shaking and I'd go over there and put blankets on him and lay on him and try to keep him warm," says Debbie. Pressure sores continued to plague him. Psychologically he wasn't doing much better. He was angry with the world, with the woman who had put him in the hospital. "I was real mad about it," he says. "She should have been watching where she was going and then I'd still be riding my motorcycle."

Like many people in this situation, Delp thought that he would walk again. When a year passed and he was still in a chair, it was another blow. "In my mind I thought it was only temporary," he says. "Debbie bought a van and put a lift in it and I got mad. Nobody could have ever told me that it was going to be permanent. I figured a couple of weeks and I'd start walking. I thought, We can always get rid of the van."

But Delp was not going to walk again. "After I got out of the hospital, I realized that I'm not going to get any better. What am I going to do? Am I just going to lay here and eat and watch TV?"

Delp is a big man, over six feet tall, broad-shouldered and barrel-chested, with close-cropped gray hair and a goatee. He loved traveling, getting outdoors, being active. And now he hated being in a wheelchair. Even more, he hated being seen in a wheelchair. After the accident, he avoided most of his old friends, a reminder of the outgoing, energetic life that he once had. He wouldn't even eat in a restaurant. Instead of going in, he'd wait in the van while Debbie picked up takeout. "I didn't want to be around somebody or see somebody that knew me and have them see me in a chair," he says. "That was a real hard thing."

And that is where most people would expect Delp's story to end, with him stuck in a wheelchair, miserable, angry, depressed, stewing over all that had been so violently taken from him. Whatever life he could build after his accident would surely not match up to the able-bodied one that he had lost: his happy and healthy retirement with nothing to do but accumulate motorized toys, travel with his wife, and indulge in the pursuits that he enjoyed. He had lost a lot, and he had every right to be upset about it. Perhaps Delp would be left with lingering post-traumatic stress symptoms such as anxiety, depression, insomnia, or even full-blown post-traumatic stress disorder. For decades nearly all of the psychological research into trauma and recovery focused on the debilitating problems that people like Delp can face—anger, guilt, hypervigilance, emotional numbness, flashbacks, even suicidal impulses that can last for years. Trauma survivors like Delp suffer through psychological pain every bit as terrible and challenging as the physical pain they must face. And that is the story that everyone is the most familiar with.

But something different happened with Delp. Despite his depression and bitterness, he continued to work at his rehabilitation, exercising and lifting weights. One evening while Delp was working out, one of the staff members at Brooks Rehabilitation, where Delp did his physical therapy, encouraged Debbie to take her husband bowling—it was a program sponsored by Brooks just for patients like Delp. Debbie brought it up, but Delp had no interest. Going out in public in his chair and trying something new, challenging, and likely awkward was a perfect combination of everything he had been avoiding since his accident. "He didn't want to go," she says. "So I got him dressed and got him in his chair and he'd say, 'Well, I'm not going out.' And I'd say, 'That's fine,' and I'd just humor him and get him out." Once in the van, Delp agreed to go in, but just to watch. Then he rolled into the bowling alley and saw two dozen people bowling, talking, laughing, and having a good time. Most of them were in wheelchairs. Debbie got him a bowling ball and wheeled him next to a man with no arms who pushed his ball with a stick held up to his chin. The person on the other side of Delp had no hands. With little choice, Delp wheeled himself up to the line across the end of the lane, picked up the ball from his lap, and rolled it toward the pins. He started to talk to the people around him. He bowled some more. He stayed all evening.

In the van on the way home, he started laughing. When Debbie asked what was so funny, he told her, "You know, the reason I didn't want to come here was that I didn't want to be around a bunch of handicapped people," he says. "Somehow I didn't realize that I was going to be one of them." That realization changed Delp. He had just found his community. The programs at Brooks and the people he met there would change his perspective on his life, and his own understanding of what he had to offer the world. "I feel normal because I can help these people. I have the use of my hands. Some people can't feed themselves," says Delp. "I think that helped me get out of the depression more than anything else."

Delp began volunteering at both the hospital and the rehabilitation center. He started talking to new spinal cord injury patients about what to expect, how the injury would change their lives, even how to manage basic things like bodily functions that would become complicated. Sometimes he's on the phone until two o'clock in the morning with friends who are wheelchair-bound. He began giving talks to college students to recruit interns for Brooks from a nearby university. "Before I got hurt, I would never have gotten up in front of a bunch of people and talked. Now I look forward to it," says Delp. "To go up to someone's hospital room, I never would have done stuff like that. I hated going to the hospital. I don't feel sorry for myself anymore."

Davis has marveled at the changes in her old friend. "He's not the same person that we knew," she says. "He's found a new way of life, of wanting to help others who are less fortunate than him." She says that before, he was outgoing, a fun and active person, but never the center of attention. He would have never considered getting up in front of people to discuss serious topics; he just wasn't confident that he had anything to offer others. His identity was the fun-loving, active, outgoing guy who just soaked up life. But that has all changed. Delp isn't happy in the same way that he used to be. "It's a different type of fulfillment that he's getting now," she says. "Materialistic things have gone away and now he is giving of himself; the true love, the true happiness that he is making others feel is where he is coming from."

Delp leads a full and meaningful life. He participates in several activities a day, everything from archery and skeet shooting to horseback riding or playing pool. He visits with patients, and helps to keep people motivated and engaged in the rehab center. He encourages people to get out to gatherings like the bowling night, and even gives some of them rides when they need it. He also lifts weights and swims to keep himself in shape so he can be as active as possible. "My life changed that day," Delp said of the accident. "I had a good life then, but I have a great life now."

How could such a horrific accident with permanent, life-altering consequences transform a good life into a profoundly better and more meaningful one? Based on the conventional wisdom about trauma, Delp should have been left broken by his experience. But instead it transformed him. He left behind a happy life brimming with leisure and fun for a new life. Now he uses his time to help others. He finds meaning in his experiences and deeper value in his friendships. His life is different; he is different. He's a person that he could never have imagined the day before he was hit by that car.

It is only in the last thirty or so years that a handful of psychologists even began asking how this could be possible, how trauma could change a person so deeply. How could it upend everything someone knew about himself and force him to build his life and sense of self anew? How could someone come out the other side of such a terrible event better, wiser, and more fulfilled? Oddly enough, the ones who first delved into this topic, who gave the phenomenon a name, started out by looking at something else entirely.

One winter day in the early 1980s, two psychology professors from the University of North Carolina at Charlotte, Richard Tedeschi and Lawrence Calhoun, drove to Atlanta, Georgia, for a conference. Calhoun had been a tenured professor for some time and Tedeschi was going to receive tenure soon. And with that promotion would come a certain amount of freedom. The door was open for each of them to pursue research projects that were a little more unorthodox, ones that they just found interesting.

Calhoun is wiry and energetic. He has a bounce to his voice and an earnest, almost boyish enthusiasm about him. For most of his career he had studied how people respond to adversity in one form or another; his work included helping people overcome various life crises. It was something that had always interested him. "I was never interested in long-term psychotherapy," says Calhoun. "I wanted short-term solutions; I wanted to work with people who were not psychotic, with whom I could make a difference and I could see that difference right away." About the time that Tedeschi got tenure, Calhoun's research partner left and he was looking for someone new to work with.

Tedeschi is a sober counterpoint to Calhoun's animated personality. He's thoughtful and soft-spoken with a neatly trimmed moustache and a full head of graying hair. He fits just about anyone's preconceived notion of a psychologist. It's easy to imagine him saying in an even and unbiased tone, "So how does that make you feel?" This slightly odd pair got along well and, more important, they had similar interests. Tedeschi was also looking for a new focus in his work, something not centered on pathologies like depression or anxiety. Over the course of the four-hour drive, they began talking about the possibility of working together and what they might study. "Wouldn't it be really interesting to talk to old people and just ask them, 'What have you learned about life that is useful, that you'd like to pass on to others?'" Calhoun remembers one of them saying. It wasn't long before they started doing just that.

They began their research by speaking to a group of widows. They didn't have elaborate questionnaires or psychological scales or models. They just asked open-ended questions and listened to what their subjects had to say. The women, who were between about fifty and eighty years old, mourned the loss of their husbands. Many of them cried nightly. Calhoun still remembers one woman who said she would wake in the middle of the night thinking she had just heard her husband put his key in the door. Then she would realize that he was gone and she'd cry all over again. But, at the same time, they told the researchers that their husbands' deaths pushed them to discover how strong they could be. Some got together with friends more often, others grew much closer to their children. Some who had never driven a car got a driver's license and gained a new independence.

Next Tedeschi and Calhoun began to speak with people who had been disabled through an accident or illness. One woman they met had become an advocate for disabled rights and saw her disability as an opportunity to find a new focus and to help others. Another person they met was a former musician and drug abuser who had been paralyzed from the waist down in a car accident. They were surprised by his attitude.

"He was not saying, 'It shattered me; I'm depressed and a shell of my former self,'" Calhoun says. Quite the opposite. While the musician was in the hospital, his doctor suggested he speak to some of the other patients who had been paralyzed and were struggling with their situation. "He found some satisfaction from that," says Tedeschi. "It ultimately became his life's work." The man went back to school, got a master's degree, and started running a rehabilitation center for people with disabilities. In the opening of their first book on this phenomenon, Tedeschi and Calhoun quote the man as saying the accident "was the one thing that happened in my life that I needed to have happen; it was probably the best thing that ever happened to me. . . . If I hadn't experienced this and lived through it, I likely wouldn't be here today. . . . If I had it to do all over again, I would want it to happen the same way."

The pair combed through psychology journals looking for other studies that might confirm their findings and provide some context for the positive changes they were recording. It was unforgiving work—they were looking for a phenomenon without a name. But bit by bit they came across a study here and there that validated what they were hearing. It was, Calhoun says, a bit like panning for gold.

One study they discovered was by a psychiatrist named William Sledge. Now a professor at the Yale School of Medicine and medical director of Yale–New Haven Psychiatric Hospital, Sledge conducted a study of aviators captured during the Vietnam War. In the mid to late 1970s, after the Vietnam War was over, Sledge was a young psychiatrist in the U.S. Air Force who was assigned to evaluate the air force aviators who had been held by the North Vietnamese in horrific conditions at the prison nicknamed the Hanoi Hilton and other locations. United States senator John McCain was held there, as was Admiral James Stockdale. Sledge had access to their entire classified debriefings so before he even met them he knew in great detail what these men had been through. Some had been held in tiny cells in solitary confinement for years; others were chained together. They were beaten and tortured, deprived of food and medical care.

When Sledge began talking to these men, he was startled by what he heard. "At first I thought I had cotton in my ears or something. The things they told me didn't make much sense," says Sledge. "They had a hard time, they were clear about that. But so often they would say things like, 'I kind of miss it. It was an intense experience. I learned a lot from it.'"

Sledge was no stranger to the idea that adversity can push a person to be stronger or more resilient. He grew up in the Deep South. His father was an attorney, so his family was relatively well-off, but the people he knew in his small town worked incredibly hard in very demanding circumstances. "There was a lot of tragedy, death, illness, alcoholism," he says. "There was an idea that if you can get through life's challenges with some grace and dignity, you would probably learn something from it. In my mind that wasn't a psychological issue; that was just human nature." But the things these prisoners of war had survived were so harsh, he had a hard time understanding how these men could take away anything positive from the experience.

He wanted to conduct a study to learn more. The air force provided him with contacts for veterans who matched his POWs almost exactly in terms of age, rank, and time spent in Southeast Asia. The only difference was that these men had never been captured. They were a perfect control group against which he could compare the POWs.

In the fall of 1976 Sledge mailed both groups questionnaires that asked about the problems they had faced in captivity or during their tour of duty, problems they faced when they returned home, and any perceived benefits and perceived problems that arose from their wartime experience, among other things.

When the questionnaires were returned Sledge found support for everything these men had been telling him in their follow-up interviews. Sixty-one percent of the POWs indicated that they had undergone beneficial changes as a result of their captivity. Only 30 percent of the control group reported this. In addition, the POWs who were held the longest and received the harshest treatment were far more likely to report positive changes than those who were held for shorter periods of time. Those who reported benefits were more optimistic, had more insight into themselves and their motivations, were better able to discern what was important in life, and felt that they got along better with others. Some even said that they enjoyed life more after their confinement. They were finding real benefits several years after they had been released.

Some of the changes make sense, Sledge says, given who these airmen were. The prisoners were the best of the best: fighter pilots and copilots. They were smart, well educated, brash, young, and filled with bravado, hardly people prone to introspection. The captivity, deprivation, and abuse forced them to spend years with little to do but reflect and to do so with the threat of death hanging over their heads. "These were people who were not used to thinking about themselves or reflecting or being introspective and now they are in a prison cell where they won't see another person with hours and hours to just sit there and think," says Sledge. "They learned to value their imagination."

One of the things that may have helped these young men was their strong sense of camaraderie. Many of the prisoners were isolated from each other in separate cells. However, they managed to communicate using a complex system of taps on cell walls, similar to Morse code. Other prisoners were chained together and locked in a cell. They were forced to gain an intimate and deep understanding of each other. "They shared their hopes about what it would be like when they got back; they talked about their families and gave each other advice. It was just an extraordinarily intense experience," says Sledge.

In 1980, Sledge's paper on the study was published. Some in the field thought it would turn heads and cause researchers to rethink their emerging understanding of the onslaught of cases of PTSD plaguing Vietnam War veterans. Sledge remembers being paired with some of the country's top trauma researchers for a panel discussion at a conference. The organizers had booked an auditorium that seated three hundred. When the discussion started, Sledge looked up to see about fifteen people in the cavernous room. And half of those were veterans. His fellow psychiatrists showed little interest in his findings. Sledge went on to other pursuits and assumed his research on the subject had been passed over.

Sledge's study might have disappeared in the stacks were it not for Tedeschi and Calhoun. For them, this study was one of those rare nuggets of gold—a published paper that confirmed they were on the right track. "It was part of a cluster of studies that had observed this phenomenon," Calhoun says of the Sledge study. "And it was amazingly influential because it allowed us to have a bit more confidence that we had identified something that really existed that other people had found in other contexts. It gave us a little more foundation to go on, so we could look forward and see what we needed to do next."

Like Sledge, Tedeschi and Calhoun are clinicians. They have had scores of patients who have been through traumatic experiences. And through their long talks with these people, they heard many of the same things that Sledge had heard from the POWs, sentiments that mirrored the responses to their open-ended research questions: events that were outwardly bad, even horrific, had spurred these survivors toward positive life changes.

As they spoke to more and more people, they began to see that traumatic experiences certainly did cause suffering, but suffering was not the end of the change wrought by these events. Suffering, in fact, was part of a much larger experience. It proved to be a kind of catalyst that pushed people to find new meaning in their lives. Tedeschi and Calhoun began to do more targeted research to discover how, exactly, these people were changing. As they dug through the existing research and interviewed more than six hundred trauma survivors, patterns began to emerge. They started correlating those responses, grouping like ones with others. Eventually they determined that people were reporting positive change in one or more of the following five distinct areas as a result of their trauma:

1. Increased inner strength
2. An openness to new possibilities in life
3. Closer and often deeper relationships with friends and family
4. An enhanced appreciation for life
5. A stronger sense of spirituality

Tedeschi and Calhoun were able to discover this phenomenon and to uncover its manifestations in large part because they took a very different approach to their work than other researchers at the time. "We were thinking in terms of what it's like for a person who's confronted with something that blows them out of the water and how can we understand that, given what we know as clinicians. That makes our thinking rare," says Calhoun. "Some of the people I have talked to who do research on these things don't spend time with people in the therapeutic context. They don't talk to people, they assess them."

Their first paper detailing these positive changes was published in 1989 and focused on the experience of the widows they spoke to. It was published in a journal that specialized in the kind of qualitative research they were using—open-ended questions much like a journalist would ask. At the same time, they realized that this approach would take them only so far. In order to spark research by other psychologists and to be accepted by the larger community of trauma researchers, they would need to be able to quantify the changes they were uncovering. Based largely on what they heard from these trauma survivors, they started to develop a standardized questionnaire designed to calculate how much of each type of change individuals reported.

But Tedeschi and Calhoun had yet to come up with a name for the phenomenon or for this new quantitative scale. They had taken to calling their new questionnaire the perceived benefits scale. "But that was such a lame name," says Calhoun. The pair bounced different ideas off one another running back and forth between their tiny offices in the psychology building at UNC Charlotte. Finally, one day, Tedeschi poked his head into Calhoun's office. "He had written a long name: blah blah blah blah blah, post-traumatic growth," Calhoun recalls. "I took one look at that and said, 'Dude, that is it.'"

Their Posttraumatic Growth Inventory, first published in a journal in 1996, asks subjects to respond to statements linked to each of the five areas of growth. They rate each of the statements on a scale between zero (there was no change) and five (I underwent a lot of change because of the crisis) so the degree of change can be measured. The statements are simple and direct, for example, "I developed new interests," or "I have a stronger religious faith."

As they conducted research and reviewed the research of others, they found to their surprise that experiencing growth in the wake of trauma is remarkably common. Half or more of all trauma survivors reported some positive changes. Growth, it turns out, is actually more common than the much better known and far better studied post-traumatic stress disorder, which researchers believe will affect about 8 percent of Americans in their lifetime and as much as 30 percent of certain groups like Vietnam War veterans.

This kind of growth, the kind that can dramatically alter a life for the better, does not occur as a result of just any upsetting event. What is required is what Tedeschi calls a seismic event—a trauma that shakes you to your core, like the accident that paralyzed Delp and left him fundamentally changed. "Growth is a rethinking, a reassessment of yourself and the world. You don't need to go through that if everything still makes sense to you," Tedeschi says. "If a person is like a building built to a high standard to withstand an earthquake, if the quake comes and the building is still standing, you are okay. But if the building suffers damage, it has to be rebuilt and the rebuilding is the growth."

Not everyone grows from traumatic experiences. But those who do are able to see that the horror and misery of trauma also create the opening for change, just as Delp saw that he had an opportunity to create a whole new way of living after his old life was stripped away by the accident and his paralysis. "The challenge is to see the opportunity presented by this seismic event. In the aftermath of the earthquake, why not build something better? Don't just live beneath the rubble, don't just build the same crappy building that you had before," says Tedeschi. "I think we can do better than that."

On a Friday evening in Jacksonville, Luther and Debbie Delp drove in their van to Bowl America, a large bowling alley in a strip mall alongside a busy four-lane road. Inside about twenty-five or thirty people took up about half of the lanes. Some people were in wheelchairs, some were in motorized chairs, some walked with crutches, and others moved slowly and stiffly with the help of a friend. Delp reached out and shook hands with each person he passed by, stopping to catch up or crack a joke. He knew just about everyone there. He wheeled himself down the ramp to the bowling lanes with a thirteen-pound ball in his lap. He stopped for a moment to talk with a mother of two children who both have spina bifida and were there bowling. (Those who can't hold a ball were using a metal track on stilts with a ramp for the ball to roll down, built by Delp's friend for the bowling alley.) Delp wheeled himself over to his lane, where he greeted a man with Parkinson's and his wife—the Delps were planning to spend a few weeks with the couple in their cabin in Maine over the summer. Bowling next to Delp was a young man who had crashed his car into a guardrail on the way to work and suffered a severe brain injury. The fact that he was up and walking and able to hold the ball was incredible, said Delp. Pointing to the person bowling on the other side of him, Delp said, "When I saw this guy in the hospital he couldn't even move a finger. He fell off a roof." Now he was up and bowling.

Another close friend, Chuck Frank, who had a stroke in 2011, was bowling with Delp. "You don't know how many people he has helped out, driving people, picking them up and dropping them off, helping them with everything," Frank said. His friendship with Delp has helped him enormously as he struggles with the debilitating aftereffects of the stroke. "He gets me laughing about a lot of things," Frank said. "Here's a guy who lost so much and he goes out and does more than me—I can't keep up with him."

After bowling, a group of about twenty drove to a nearby diner where a band was playing in the parking lot and a few dozen classic cars were on display. Delp wheeled around the lot, checking out the cars' gleaming engines and pristine vintage interiors while talking with friends over the loud music. Then they all went inside for dinner. The group took up four or five tables at the back of the fifties-themed diner. Everyone was talking and eating and having a great time. Delp was sitting at a table in the middle of the group, a club sandwich in front of him. Here, surrounded by this group of new friends, people he never would have known before his life-changing accident, he smiled, looking happy, like he belonged.

Delp's dramatic transformation is exactly what Tedeschi and Calhoun have been studying all these years—someone who has re-invented himself after a terrible event, someone who has found new meaning and value in his life. And he is also someone they hope their research will help. "The ability to say, 'There's a name for these things I have been experiencing or the way I have been thinking about this,' is important," says Calhoun. "Hopefully we have captured what these people have experienced, and now they know what it is."

The basic principles that Tedeschi and Calhoun laid out in their first book and the inventory they developed to track growth have proven to be remarkably accurate. They and the legions of researchers who have followed have been able to learn more about the nuances of growth, how it works, who is likely to grow, and what can help to facilitate it, without doing much revision to the original theory. "Part of why it's stood the test of time is because we just listened to people who had gone through these events," says Tedeschi. "We let them teach us. We didn't come at this as people who consider themselves experts in the field. We knew we had a lot to learn. We were curious about it. And to a great degree we just put the scientific shine on the stories of people that we had been talking to. The theories evolved out of that work, which is why it worked out so well."

In the two decades since Tedeschi and Calhoun published their first book on post-traumatic growth, researchers around the world have begun examining the phenomenon. Psychologists in China, Japan, Turkey, Iran, Italy, England, Australia, Israel, and other countries have conducted studies examining growth. They have studied cancer survivors and their spouses, prisoners of war, immigrants, survivors of natural disaster, and more. And over and over they are finding that more than half of trauma survivors grow. Growth seems to be a widespread phenomenon—in the experience of trauma survivors everywhere, and even in the stories, old and new, told in cultures around the world.

CHAPTER 2

The Psychiatrist in the Death Camp

From Modern Psychology to Popular Culture,
Post-Traumatic Growth Is Everywhere

TEDESCHI AND CALHOUN WORK IN AN UNGLAMOROUS, BOXY,
1960s brick classroom building that houses the University of North
Carolina at Charlotte's psychology department. On a winter morning, a meeting of their research team composed of graduate students
was held in a windowless classroom full of empty desks—Tedeschi
forgot to sign up for the "nice room," said Calhoun. One student
discussed a research project involving computerized surveys in great
detail only to be reminded that the computers in the lab were un-
available because of a renovation that had already taken two years.

Despite the years of groundbreaking work Tedeschi and Calhoun
have conducted, they have not seen a deluge of funding. Yet the situation is far better than it once was. "When we started out [funding]
was nonexistent; even getting anything published was hard," Tedeschi
says. When they began their work, Tedeschi and Calhoun were pushing back against the mainstream of thought in psychology. No one
wanted to hear that trauma could result in positive change. The focus

was on the dysfunction that resulted from trauma, and how to "fix" it. But this wasn't always the conventional thinking in psychological circles.

In 1942, Viktor Frankl was a successful young neurologist and psychiatrist living in Vienna. He ran the neurological department at the Jewish hospital and had been married just a year earlier. But in September of that year, he and his wife were arrested by Nazi soldiers. His family was rounded up and Frankl, his wife, and his parents were loaded onto a train and sent to the Theresienstadt concentration camp, in what is now the Czech Republic. In the fall of 1944 he and his wife and mother were loaded onto another train. This time they were taken to Auschwitz. Frankl was quickly separated from his family and was moved again. All of his family members died in the camps, yet somehow Frankl survived. The years of unimaginable suffering, misery, and fear changed Frankl, but perhaps not in the way one would imagine.

In his book *Man's Search for Meaning*, written just months after the end of the war, Frankl tells of the horrors of life in the camp, how the Nazis systematically dehumanized each prisoner, beating them, working them until nothing was left, and his own struggle to survive physically and psychologically:

Under the influence of a world which no longer recognized the value of human life and human dignity, which had robbed man of his will and made him an object to be exterminated (having planned, however, to make full use of him first—to the last ounce of his physical resources)— under this influence the personal ego finally suffered a loss of values. If the man in the concentration camp did not struggle against this in a last effort to save his self-respect, he lost the feeling of being an individual, a being with a mind and inner freedom and personal value. He thought of

*himself then as only a part of an enormous mass of people; his existence
descended to the level of animal life.*

Then, one evening, almost by accident, Frankl discovered something that would save his life. As he marched back from a work detail that evening, he was in terrible pain. His feet were covered in sores, his shoes torn. With a bitterly cold wind bearing down on him, he obsessed over all the tiny things he needed to do in order to survive. If a piece of sausage were given to him, should he trade it for bread? Should he trade a cigarette he had squirreled away for a bowl of soup? How could he find a piece of wire to replace the bit that had served as a shoelace? How could he get on good terms with the guard who might be able to assign him to a closer work detail? Then, in the midst of this complex calculus of survival, an image came to him. He saw a detailed and clear vision of himself giving a lecture after the war on the psychology of the concentration camp. And that changed how he viewed everything around him. "All that oppressed me at that moment became objective, seen as described from the remote viewpoint of science. By this method I succeeded in rising above the situation, above the sufferings of the moment," he wrote.

He also thought about his wife. His love for her grew, helped to sustain him, to give him some meaning as he struggled to survive day to day, hour to hour. He thought a lot about inner life, about dignity and conduct. He remembered Nietzsche, who wrote, "He who has a *why* to live can bear with almost any *how*." It was not just a call to find meaning, but a demand. Meaning was not a luxury for Frankl. It was the difference between life and death.

In *Man's Search for Meaning*, which has sold more than 10 million copies since its publication in 1946, Frankl lays out a way of thinking about suffering, trauma, and the psychological aftereffects that is totally at odds with how modern psychology views pathology. For Frankl, the suffering that can result from trauma—depression, anxiety, and many of the other symptoms—are not always maladies to be cured, like a sore throat or a broken leg. Instead they can be important indications of inner turmoil. They are normal. More than that, he says, they are an achievement. These problems demand atten-tion and will only be cured in the course of resolving the underlying inner conflict. In many cases, treating the symptom only prolongs the disease in his view. He writes that

suffering is not always a pathological phenomenon; rather than being a symptom of neurosis, suffering may well be a human achievement, especially if the suffering grows out of existential frustration. I would strictly deny that one's search for meaning to his existence, or even his doubt of it, in every case is derived from, or results in, any disease. Existential frustration is in itself neither pathological nor pathogenic. A man's concern, even his despair, over the worthwhileness of life is an existential distress but by no means a mental disease. It may well be that interpreting the first in terms of the latter motivates a doctor to bury his patient's existential despair under a heap of tranquilizing drugs. It is his task, rather, to pilot the patient through his existential crisis of growth and development.

Frankl went on to found an entire branch of psychotherapy fo-cused on the idea of finding meaning in one's life, and particularly in one's suffering. He called this *logotherapy*, and he focused on meaning as the central driving force of a healthy life.

Just a few years before Frankl's book was published, an American psychologist, Abraham Maslow, published a paper laying out his concept of the hierarchy of needs. Human beings, he argued, are motivated by increasing their well-being and are on a trajectory toward self-actualization, which included attributes like morality, creativity, and problem solving. Maslow studied the life stories of some of the highest achievers: Albert Einstein, Frederick Douglass, Eleanor Roosevelt. When studying these successful figures, Maslow found that their most important learning experiences were often the tragedies and traumas that force people to take a new perspective on life.

From the 1940s onward, Maslow was one of a group of humanistic psychologists who studied and pushed for more examination of flourishing. "They were disenchanted with the focus of the field of psychology, which was interested in what was wrong with people instead of trying to understand human potential," says Louis Hoffman, a faculty member at Saybrook University—a San Francisco school founded by a group of humanistic psychologists in 1971.

But by the 1980s, humanistic psychology was starting to fall out of favor. The field, which had always maintained its focus on pathology even at the height of interest in the humanistic psychologists, began to shift away from its brief flirtation with flourishing. One contributing factor was likely the Vietnam War. Many soldiers returning from battle were having severe mental health problems. While today *post-traumatic stress disorder* is a common term, it was not even recognized as a diagnosis until 1980, when it was first included in the *Diagnostic and Statistical Manual of Mental Disorders* (or *DSM*), the bible of mental-health diagnosis. But of course soldiers have been telling tales of the horrific aftereffects of battle as long as people have been recording history. In Homer's *Iliad*, written in the eighth century B.C., Achilles is racked by pain and anger at the death of his friend Patroclus. Soldiers in the American Civil War were said to suffer from soldier's heart. In World War I it was shell shock, and in World War II it was battle fatigue.

Because of the unique way that the brain processes traumatic events, memories of these horrific events can be triggered by all kinds of sounds, smells, and experiences. And when that memory is triggered, the body and brain react as if the person were once again in the thick of the trauma, fighting once more for their lives. These memories are exhausting and overwhelming and can leave a person depressed, anxious, and unable to function and can cause self-destructive, even suicidal behavior.

Trauma and the damaging aftereffects are not limited to experiences on the battlefield. Losing a loved one suddenly, surviving cancer or other life-threatening medical conditions, experiencing natural disasters or terrorist attacks, being the victim of a violent or sexual assault, even severe financial or career loss can be traumatic. Researchers estimate that about 75 percent of people will experience a traumatic event in their lifetime.

In the 1980s, Stephen Joseph, then a graduate student in psychology from Northern Ireland, began his own research into trauma by examining the experiences of the survivors of a passenger ship disaster. On a spring night in 1987, the *Herald of Free Enterprise*, a passenger ferry, pulled out of port in Belgium, bound for England. The bow door had not been properly secured and almost immediately the ship began to take on water. When the captain attempted to turn the ship, it rolled on its side. Water flooded the passenger compartment. Electricity went out. "Some people were trapped for hours in the dark in icy water. Dead bodies floated around them," Joseph says. "It was absolutely horrific." Of the nearly six hundred passengers and crew, 193 people died. Joseph spent the next three years studying the survivors and their reactions to the trauma.

Joseph focused on the survivors' struggles: depression, PTSD, alcohol and drug use, survivor's guilt, and anxiety. But in his conversations with survivors, he noticed something else. Many of them spoke about positive changes in their lives, too. Joseph was not entirely surprised to hear this. Post-traumatic stress disorder was a relatively new idea in the 1980s. Joseph had a background in social psychology and many in that field had identified something called positive reframing—applying a positive meaning to negative events as a means of coping with it. Social psychologists saw such reframing as a tool that people used to help manage difficult experiences.

Joseph was interested in discovering how positive reframing was working in those who survived the disaster. In his survey he included a single question about whether the survivor's view of life had changed in a positive way or a negative way in the three years since the disaster. Though he expected some positive responses, he was amazed by the results: 43 percent said their view of life had changed for the better. Most wrote that they valued relationships and other people more, that they now lived life to its fullest, that they had more empathy, even that they were more driven to succeed.

"Listening to people talk about these things, it was life changing for me as a young man setting out on a career," says Joseph. "As a psychologist, it was a turning point in my life. The way people came out of this, in a way that was transformative even though many of them were still struggling with post-traumatic stress symptoms, it shaped what I was looking for." Joseph started to think that this positive reframing might not be just a coping mechanism. Instead, something bigger and more profound might have resulted from the trauma—shifts in personality, in a person's entire outlook on life. Joseph's work with the survivors of the ferry disaster sparked his interest in the humanistic psychologists. Their ideas about growth and positive life change resonated with his own experience even as those very ideas were falling out of favor with most psychologists.

Joseph went on to become a psychology professor at the University of Nottingham in England and, alongside Tedeschi and Calhoun, is one of the most important early researchers on post-traumatic growth, publishing dozens of studies, working as a clinician with trauma survivors, and writing a book about growth, titled *What Doesn't Kill Us*. Throughout his career he has worked to apply the basic tenets of the humanistic psychologists to modern themes, keeping their work relevant, incorporating their approaches and interest in flourishing and meaning into his own work.

In the 1990s, Martin Seligman, a professor at the University of Pennsylvania, and other psychologists began looking at some of those same themes: What made great people great? What is happiness and how do we achieve it? When Seligman was elected president of the American Psychological Association in 1998, he was given a rare opportunity to push his ideas into the mainstream of psychology. Seligman chose to make positive psychology the theme of his tenure as president. He has gone on to author many books on the subject, including the bestseller *Authentic Happiness*.

Seligman loves to tell a good story and can entertain a crowd in a way that is rare among academics. And he can be a relentless promoter. In person he spins tales with heartfelt enthusiasm about rubbing elbows with politicians and high-level military figures. One psychologist, who asked not to be named since Seligman is a powerful figure, said Seligman is to positive psychology what P. T. Barnum was to circuses.

While that may be a slight to an academic, in a way that was just what positive psychology, and indeed the entire endeavor of looking at positive change, needed: a P. T. Barnum. It needed a booster, a promoter, a salesman, because it was looking to turn the focus of an entire field in the opposite direction. Psychology has long focused on understanding human behavior and mental processes and, primarily, helping those in distress—diagnosing mental illnesses like depression and working to help people regain their mental health. But Seligman thought that psychology could do much more than that—it could not just help to pull people up from the depths of despair to some baseline of functionality, but it could actually help everyone lead better lives, orienting people, and perhaps even society, toward positive change and achievement.

Positive psychology is not necessarily concerned with post-traumatic growth, though some of its adherents have contributed to its study. But positive psychology reopened the door to the whole idea of examining and promoting positive change. In a field steeped in pathology, those researching post-traumatic growth suddenly found themselves with powerful allies who were looking for positive changes everywhere. "Positive psychology has been a tremendously successful vehicle," says Joseph. "Positive psychology and post-traumatic growth have helped to bring those humanistic ideas back to the fore, into contemporary psychology. It has been a tremendous achievement."

Tedeschi, Calhoun, and others delving into post-traumatic growth have faced skeptics from the beginning. Growth sounded too good to be true. It didn't align well with the dominant theory of trauma: that people went through an experience, exhibited some post-traumatic stress symptoms, and then over time returned to normal, except for the few that were plagued by PTSD.

Some, like Howard Tennen, a professor at the University of Connecticut, thought that growth might actually be real, but Tennen had problems with the way it is measured. All of the research on post-traumatic growth asks people to assess how they have changed after the traumatic event takes place. But that can be problematic. Psychologists are asking people to assess their own changes after the fact. They could simply be wrong, perhaps inventing the growth as a means of justifying the trauma and symptoms they have survived. The best way to understand how trauma changes a person would be to avoid asking individuals to make that assessment at all. Instead a psychologist taking the best approach would assess the individual prior to a traumatic event to establish a baseline, and then assess the individual again after the event. Then researchers could compare the two objective assessments to determine what, if anything, had changed without ever asking the individual for his own opinion about how he had changed. The obvious problem with doing such a study is that it is very hard to find people who will go through a traumatic event during the course of the research. A psychologist could contact ten thousand people and over the course of a year or two, maybe only a few would have gone through something traumatic— hardly enough cases to base a study on. These studies were not really practical.

So, just about all the research on post-traumatic growth asks people to make their own assessment about how the trauma has changed them after the trauma has occurred. Tennen says the psychological literature shows that people are unreliable when it comes to assessing how much they have changed. "I have no doubt that there are people, perhaps many people, who do change in positive ways, but we are not able to conceptualize and measure it," Tennen says.

Tedeschi, Calhoun, and many others in the field agree that the research could be stronger, and better research would only help psychologists to understand more about the phenomenon. But they are also adamant that post-traumatic growth is real and can be measured.

"Virtually all psychological research relies on memory," says Tedeschi. "If you decide that memory is unreliable then you have to throw out everything that has ever been published in psychology."

Several studies have tried to address these shortcomings. In 2008, Jane Shakespeare-Finch, an associate professor at the Queensland University of Technology in Brisbane, Australia, surveyed a group of sixty-one trauma survivors using the Posttraumatic Growth Inventory. She then asked a family member to assess their loved one's changes using the same inventory. She found that the positive changes reported by the trauma survivors were corroborated by the family member.

One long-term study, begun by the U.S. Army in 2008, may eventually put this debate to rest for good. Researchers selected five hundred soldiers before they deployed to Iraq and surveyed them to assess their baseline. They surveyed them while in combat, and again about six weeks after they returned home, and once again a year and a half after they returned from combat, and they plan to contact them again later. Though the study is not yet complete, Colonel Patrick Sweeney, who was at the U.S. Military Academy at West Point when the study began and is now at Wake Forest University, says that more than half of the soldiers he interviewed after their deployment who were exposed to potentially traumatic battlefield events had experienced some type of growth. They reported having a greater sense of confidence in their abilities, a greater appreciation for life, and a stronger sense of priorities. The study is already turning up the kind of objective data on growth that may well show even the most scrupulous critic that growth is not just real but can be measured, examined, and understood.

•   •   •

Some researchers say that growth, or the perception of growth, might be influenced by culture. Americans in particular are bombarded with so many messages about the need to learn from and benefit from adverse experiences that trauma survivors here might be telling themselves that they have grown in order to conform to a cultural norm. People are certainly influenced by the culture around them. And stories of post-traumatic growth are everywhere from ancient history to religion, in the lives of our most celebrated people and even in popular culture. Everyone has been exposed to these tales. They are some of our best-known and most powerful stories.

One of the most succinctly rendered and best-known stories of post-traumatic growth first appeared in 1939. It was only two illustrated pages long and told the story of a young boy who watches as his parents are senselessly murdered by a robber. Then, just days later, the boy is shown at his bedside offering this prayer: "I swear by the spirits of my parents to avenge their deaths by spending the rest of my life warring on all criminals."

The young boy, of course, is Bruce Wayne, and he takes on the character of the superhero Batman to fight crime and protect the city of Gotham at all costs. As depicted in that early comic strip, he is transformed—almost instantly—by the brutal murder of his parents. He is motivated to become a "master scientist," to become physically powerful, and to dedicate his life and his sizable fortune to a broader altruistic cause: fighting crime and protecting others.

For those who worked on the series for more than seventy years after it was conceived, it was clear that this story moved readers and tapped some fundamental experience that fans easily identified with. Dennis O'Neil, who edited the series on and off between the 1970s and 2000, was given the chance to change Batman's origin story. "I said no," he says. "In this one sentence—Batman saw his parents murdered when he was a child—we have everything we need to know about him. His motivation is literal. Everything is perfect."

Batman isn't the only superhero who is transformed by loss. Peter Parker in the *Spider-Man* series begins using his powers to fight evil only after the tragic death of his uncle. The Green Lantern witnesses the death of his own father in a plane crash. The Flash's mother was murdered. Loss and transformation is a constant theme.

Despite the superpowers and fantastical story lines in these comics, those who developed the stories of these superheroes were inspired by real people. Paul Levitz, who wrote and edited for DC Comics for forty-two years and was its president from 2002 until 2009, had an outsize role in shaping the stories of American popular culture. And for him, the tale of post-traumatic growth was not only an engaging one that connected with readers; it was fundamentally grounded in the story of another well-known American: Teddy Roosevelt.

Roosevelt was born into a powerful and wealthy family, but as a child he suffered from severe asthma, which left him confined indoors for much of his childhood. He developed an especially close relationship with his father, who often stayed up late at night with him when he was sick. When Roosevelt was in college, his father died suddenly of cancer, which he'd hidden from the family. As a way of honoring his father, Roosevelt dedicated himself to public service, an unusual choice for a wealthy young man at the time. Roosevelt was driven to achieve. By the age of twenty-four he was already a New York State assemblyman. Two and a half years later, in February 1884, his first daughter, Alice, was born.

Then, just two days later, tragedy struck. Roosevelt's wife and his mother died within hours of each other.

The young man was shattered, writing in his journal, "The light has gone out of my life." Roosevelt withdrew from public life, left his infant daughter with his sister, and headed west to live on a ranch in North Dakota. He built a cabin and raised cattle. Roosevelt took off on long hunting trips where he shot grizzly bears and other big game. Sometimes he rode on horseback alone for days through blizzards and below-zero temperatures, pushing himself to physical and psychological extremes. He found a remarkable fearlessness, confronting gunmen who threatened to kill him and hunting down cattle thieves. But when he slowed down, grief would overwhelm him.

Eventually Roosevelt returned to New York and was appointed to run New York City's police commission. He took to the streets and walked officers' beats to ensure that they were doing their jobs. He exposed corruption on the force and locked horns with powerful and deeply corrupt political figures. He patrolled the city alongside muckraking journalists. Roosevelt, in his time with the commission, became a transformative force for reform, much as he would later as president.

Almost seventy years after Batman's origin was divulged in those two succinct comic book pages, Christopher Nolan, who directed the 2008 Batman film *The Dark Knight*, based parts of the film on Theodore Roosevelt's life and urged its star, Christian Bale, to read a biography of Roosevelt. Nolan found inspiration in Roosevelt's story, just like Levitz had during his career at DC Comics. It became a touchstone to shape the stories of other superheroes, stories that have helped people to understand how adversity can change them. "People succeed in wonderful and dramatic ways in history," says Levitz. "And that provides the inspiration for what the heroic journey can be."

That heroic journey—the archetype of many of our oldest stories—is at its core a story of post-traumatic growth. Joseph Campbell, who studied myths of cultures around the world, discovered common themes hidden in those stories. The archetypal myth of the hero, one of the most common stories, begins with the protagonist leaving his or her home, or at times with the destruction of a home. Then the hero is presented with a series of challenges, often traumatic or violent ones, sometimes involving a trip to the underworld. At the end of the journey he or she returns home, often avenging wrongs and becoming a changed and enlightened leader.

The theme of post-traumatic growth can be found in Homer's *Odyssey*, in the stories of the knights searching for the Holy Grail, in Dante's *Inferno*, in the four-thousand-year-old myths of the Sumerians, and in modern-day shamanistic cultures, says Evans Lansing Smith, who traveled extensively with Campbell and is now the chair of the mythological studies program at Pacifica Graduate Institute, which is home to the Joseph Campbell Collection. The theme continues through Batman to today's superheroes. The story of growth is as old as our oldest recorded history and seems to appear everywhere.

These stories of growth have certainly influenced our culture. But they are also grounded in real people's lives. Theodore Roosevelt's life experience, and the ways that loss and grief molded him, helped to inform the stories of comic book characters for decades. And those characters in turn influenced the way that everyday people think about adversity, change, and their own potential. So, certainly people are influenced by their culture and do develop expectations about how they should react to trauma. But that culture is also influenced by real-life figures who go through real psychological processes. They grow because people often do grow. And the stories that result reflect that. Our myths are not made of fantasy.

And, it turns out, these concepts of trauma, growth, and change are not simply a creation of Western culture. Tzipi Weiss, associate professor of social work at Long Island University's LIU Post campus, examined how culture influences post-traumatic growth in a book she coedited, *Posttraumatic Growth and Culturally Competent Practice: Lessons Learned from Around the Globe*. Weiss reviewed published studies of trauma survivors from more than a dozen different cultures. She found studies that reported post-traumatic growth in Israelis who survived terrorist attacks and Palestinians confined in Israeli prisons, in Turkish victims of earthquakes and Chinese breast cancer survivors, and in other populations around the world. "It's pretty clear that post-traumatic growth is a universal phenomenon," she says.

And perhaps that is why Tedeschi and Calhoun's work has caught on. Researchers around the globe are pursuing questions about growth from every angle in dozens of cultures. In fact, growth has become part of an entirely new way of understanding trauma, as not just a temporary setback or an illness-inducing event, but as a fundamentally transformative experience—one that changes people psychologically, and even alters the way their brains function. As Tedeschi and Calhoun theorized decades ago, researchers from an array of fields are discovering that trauma causes fundamental change. "It's pretty mind-boggling," says Calhoun of the entire field of study he and Tedeschi sparked. "We're not even Chapel Hill, let alone Harvard or Princeton. It feels very good."

CHAPTER 3

That Was Traumatic?

Neuroscience and the Personal Nature of Trauma

IN APRIL 1968, MAX CLELAND WAS A YOUNG CAPTAIN WITH THE 1st Air Cavalry Division, an all-helicopter unit, the only one of its kind in Vietnam. Cleland, the future U.S. senator from Georgia, extended his service for a year just so he could join it—he was eager to see combat. But after ten months in the country he had only been in light mortar attacks; it was not the kind of soul-testing battle experience he had somewhat naively hoped for.

Cleland had just received his discharge papers and was due to head home in a few weeks when his unit was called up as part of an offensive to help a group of five thousand marines who were surrounded by twenty thousand North Vietnamese soldiers in Khe Sanh. Cleland's commander told him that he could stay behind since he was scheduled to return home so soon, but Cleland insisted that he go. But as the date got closer, and he learned the details of the mission, the six-foot-two paratrooper began to worry. His unit was going to be dropped off on the hilltops surrounding Khe Sanh to support a large force of ground troops. But they would be within easy shot of

North Vietnamese artillery, leaving the soldiers little to do but hunker down and hope they didn't get blown up. He told his commanding officer that he'd changed his mind, that he didn't want to go. But it was too late to back out. In the days leading up to the attack, it was all he could do to manage his fear.

When Cleland looked down from the chopper as his unit was flown into position, he saw a landscape of turned-up earth, pockmarked with craters from American bombs—the result of an effort to deprive the North Vietnamese of anywhere to hide. Of course, it also deprived American soldiers of the same cover. Cleland and his fellow soldiers got off the chopper, climbed into a crater, and dug in. That first night rockets whistled as they fell all around him. The sky lit up as both sides did their best to annihilate each other. When the sun rose the next morning Cleland saw four dead soldiers from his battalion, their bodies ravaged from exploding rockets and mortar fire. The battle raged on for four days. Two hundred men from his division died, but in the end the North Vietnamese were defeated. Cleland had seen the fires of battle and come through it, and soon he would be heading home.

He and a few soldiers hopped on a chopper to pick up new communications equipment from the field base. One of them was a new guy, someone he had never seen before. When the chopper landed, Cleland was the last off. He ducked his head and ran out, past the perimeter of the chopper's swirling blades. And that's when he saw it: a grenade. It was just lying there on the ground. Cleland thought that he must have dropped it. He pushed his M-16 behind his back with his left hand and reached out to grab it with his right. Just as his outstretched fingers were about to grasp the grenade, it exploded.

He saw a flash of white. There was a powerful explosion and he was hurled through the air. He felt his eyes being pushed back into his skull. Cleland landed hard on the ground. The sound echoed through his ears. When he opened his eyes he saw a stub of broken bone where his right arm had been. One leg was gone. The other was turned completely around. His pants were soaked in blood and were smoking. He tried yelling; nothing but a hiss came out. His windpipe was torn open. If not for the fast action of medics who stanched the bleeding with tourniquets, he surely would have died. Overwhelmed by pain, Cleland was fighting for his life.

Cleland didn't know that he was in danger when he reached out for the grenade. But as he lay on the ground, blown to pieces, he knew from the faces of those looking at him, from the life he could feel ebbing from him with every beat of his heart, that death was close. He fought back, forcing himself to stay conscious as he was flown to a hospital for surgery. He did everything he could to stay awake and stay alive.

During an event like this, where someone's life is threatened, their bodies and brains go through a set of actions and reactions that are completely out of the individual's control. If, for example, a person steps into a crosswalk and then looks up to see a car coming at him, that visual information is sent to a part of the brain called the thalamus, a kind of relay station. From there it is routed in two different directions. A quick sketch of the information is sent directly to the amygdala, a part of the brain involved with emotional reactions and, crucially, the fight or flight response. At the same time a much more detailed set of information is sent to the visual cortex where a more nuanced picture of the event is assembled. When the amygdala receives the initial burst of distressing information, it triggers the hypothalamus, which begins to activate the sympathetic nervous system. Adrenaline, cortisol, and norepinephrine flood the system. At first muscles contract and the person freezes in anticipation of what's to come (remaining motionless can also be an advantageous response to danger since many predators look for movement). Then breathing rate increases, as does heart rate. Blood flow is increased to muscles. Fat is made ready for quick fuel. Pupils dilate to allow more light in. All of these changes help the individual to either fight off the perceived danger or flee it—jump out of the way of the oncoming car. It's why after a brush with immediate danger or even the appearance of danger, it's common to sweat, to breathe hard, to feel the heart racing.

At the same time, a more detailed picture of the threatening sensory information is being assembled in the visual cortex. And the contextual information—where the person is, what is happening around them—is all being combined and sent to the hippocampus. Eventually this information is transmitted to the amygdala. Part of the amygdala's function is to determine what is and is not a threat. Joseph LeDoux, a professor of neuroscience at New York University, in his most recent book, *Anxious: Using the Brain to Understand and Treat Fear and Anxiety*, writes that the associations between a stimulus and a threat (in the case of decades of lab tests, a bell or light and an electric shock) are encoded and stored in a part of the amygdala called the lateral nucleus. It uses that association between a stimulus and pain to determine what warrants the jumpstarting of the fight or flight response. By learning to associate the sound of a bell and a shock, people and animals will eventually display the fight or flight response to just the sound of the bell, whether or not the shock is administered (that same response can also be broken by exposing the subject to the sound repeatedly without any shock). Other regions of the brain that are connected to the amygdala help to determine the intensity of the response and can help to break associations between stimulus and threats.

The fight or flight response is often erroneously activated by that first initial, but undetailed, burst of information from the thalamus to the amygdala. But if that blur of the car hurtling toward the individual turns out to be slowing down or turning out of the way (something that can be determined thanks to the more detailed information from the visual cortex and other contextual information—the width of the street, or proximity to the car), the amygdala will determine that there is no threat. The fight or flight response will be turned off. With this quick burst of vague information, the body gets a jump-start on its life-saving efforts, possibly averting death or injury with quick action. Nothing is lost if it occurred in error.

The hormones released in these events cause some extreme changes and are meant to preserve life. They enable all resources to be mustered for the emergency at hand. The amygdala also communicates back to many parts of the brain during such an event, including areas associated with working and long-term memory, helping to focus attention on the immediate threat.

Many people who go through this type of trauma report that time slowed down. Cleland recalls being thrown up into the air and landing hard on the ground. He heard the sound of the explosion echoing, drowning out everything else. He felt the force of the blast pushing his eyes back into their sockets. These are all details that would seem impossible to notice in the fraction of a second in which the explosion happened.

That phenomenon has puzzled David Eagleman, a neuroscientist at the Baylor College of Medicine, ever since he fell off the roof of a home under construction when he was a young boy. Eagleman remembers thinking as he fell that this must have been what it was like for Alice when she fell down the rabbit hole. He noticed tiny details—the bricks below, the edge of the roof. When he got older, he figured out that the fall took only eight-tenths of a second—not long enough to really think of or notice anything. Why, he wondered, was this memory so vivid? Why did he perceive this fall as taking so long? Do people perceive time differently in life-threatening situations or is something else at work?

Eagleman collected more than four hundred narratives from people who survived an instantaneous life-threatening situation, and all of them described some version of time slowing down. It seemed to be a universal experience. So he and his coauthors devised an experiment that would give them some insight into what exactly happened in these situations. The subjects fell backward off a ninety-foot-tall tower into a net. As they fell they looked at a watch on their wrists that flashed information at a rate too fast for people to see. If they were perceiving time differently as they plummeted to the ground, they would be able to read the messages on the watch.

Though each subject thought the fall took longer than it actually did, none of them was able to read the blinking message on the watch. People do not experience time any differently during these life-threatening events, Eagleman and the other researchers discovered. Instead they have a very different perception of the event. "Essentially all systems are concentrated on the issue at hand," he says. "Normally the brain is involved in dozens of other activities—what you are going to have for lunch, whether your career is going well—but when you are in a life-threatening situation, an enormous amount of attention suddenly gets focused on one thing. We lay down very dense memories, all of the tiny details that usually never get encoded." When we access those memories later, they are so detailed—so much more so than any other memories we have—that our only interpretation of them is that this event must have taken a long time.

Repeated exposure to these kinds of life-threatening—or even just stressful—events actually causes measurable change in the brain. Ki Ann Goosens, an investigator at the McGovern Institute for Brain Research at the Massachusetts Institute of Technology, has been studying what fear and stress do to the brains of rats. In order to stress the animals, she puts them in a cloth tube, like the pastry tubes that chefs use for icing cakes. They are squeezed into the tube with their noses protruding so they can breathe and smell but are unable to move or see. Goosens sits the rats upright for about four hours a day. Though it doesn't harm them, the rats hate it and they get very stressed from the experience.

When she examined the brains of these rats, she found something surprising. All of the activity in the brain's fear center from daily stress changed the amygdala. The amygdala in the stressed rats was larger than the amygdala of rats who were not stressed. She also discovered a previously unknown link between stress and the hormone ghrelin. It is best known as the hormone that causes people (and rats) to feel hungry. But ghrelin also sparks growth in the amygdala. Goosens found that the body releases ghrelin as a result of stress, and that unlike cortisol and adrenaline, which the body also releases as a result of fear, the levels of ghrelin stay high for a month or more after the stressful event has passed. While her research is preliminary, she says that ghrelin, which is released due to stress, may have an impact on increased activity in the amygdala. And all of that activity in the amygdala changes how trauma survivors remember the event, even how they think and act after the trauma.

After his surgery, Cleland was sent back to Walter Reed Army Medical Center, in Washington, D.C. There he underwent more surgeries and grueling physical therapy. It is also where he found a group of officers who had suffered similarly life-altering injuries. They were all struggling with the same kinds of problems and relied on each other to get through the day. In the middle of their room, painted on the floor, was the image of a snake—they called it the snake pit. "We had all lost something," Cleland says. "We'd cry at night and help each other through the day and everyone struggled to get better. I am still in touch with some of them over forty years later. That was the most powerful support group I ever had and none of us even knew it, we just survived together."

But that support group fell apart when one by one the men were released from the hospital. At the time there was no group therapy or mental health services of any kind for wounded soldiers. They were simply sent out the door and usually started reporting to the Veterans Administration for rehabilitation.

Without his buddies from the snake pit, and all of the support and routines he had become used to at Walter Reed, Cleland became angry and bitter, at times depressed, even suicidal. He railed against himself, for volunteering for the mission that he didn't need to go on, for sloppiness that allowed the pin to fall from his grenade (he would find out years later that the grenade actually belonged to that mysterious new guy on the chopper who hadn't bent his grenade pins back to keep them in place the way soldiers were trained to do). He was angry at the army and the VA. He was obsessed with and over-whelmed by the life that he lost, the future that he always imagined that would never materialize.

Cleland had long been interested in politics and public service. But that seemed like a fantasy now. His easy athleticism was stripped from him. He would never have a girlfriend, get married, have a family. He stewed over why this happened to him. He drank. Often drinking himself to sleep was the only way he could rest. But when he did finally doze off, the nightmares were often more horrible than his waking life. In the years that followed he was convinced that he was in danger and obsessively checked his door locks and oven knobs—a sign of his growing obsessive-compulsive disorder. Eventually he suffered from a growing fear that something terrible was about to befall him and there was nothing he could do to stop it. And later in life, feelings of fear and hopelessness would flood in without warning, placing him right back in Vietnam fighting for his life.

Cleland certainly survived a traumatic event, by any definition. And, as he would learn much later, that horrific blast left him struggling not only with life-altering injuries, but also with post-traumatic stress disorder. But in 1968, PTSD was not yet recognized—it would be another twelve years before the diagnosis even found a place in the *DSM*. Since then, with the advent of brain imaging technology, researchers have learned a remarkable amount about how people respond to trauma. They are starting to understand that people don't just suffer through a traumatic event and then bounce back. Instead a trauma survivor's understanding of himself and the world around him, his identity, and even the way his brain functions can be profoundly changed by the trauma.

Most people who survive a traumatic event can eventually put the experience in context. We learn that just because we were hit by a car, not every car we see poses a mortal threat. Yet for a small percentage of trauma survivors, that does not happen. About 8 percent of Americans will experience PTSD in their lifetimes, and for combat veterans the prevalence is higher—anywhere from 10 percent to 30 percent, depending on which war they served in. For these individuals, the root of the problem is usually an overactive amygdala which, when triggered, causes many other parts of the brain to focus intently on the perceived threat. Cognitive processing systems involved in working memory and attention are engaged as are parts of the sensory cortex, causing the person to focus senses on the threat to the exclusion of other information. At the same time the systems that help people determine what is and isn't a legitimate threat—such as the hippocampus, which helps with understanding the context surrounding a potential threat—are impaired. This in turn makes it harder to turn the fight or flight response down or off, or to learn that some things no longer pose a threat at all. The ability to extinguish the association between certain stimuli and harm is also impaired. People with PTSD often avoid any situation that could remind them of the event, to avoid the flood of horrific memories and the triggering of the fight or flight response. Unfortunately, that deprives them of the opportunity to learn new contextual information that should curb that response—for example, learning that, off the battlefield, loud sounds are no longer a mortal threat.

Because of the overactive amygdala in those with PTSD, the fight or flight response is easily triggered. And that easy and unpredictable initiation of such an overwhelming reaction causes severe anxiety. That anxiety causes further arousal of the amygdala. The more one reacts, the more anxious one becomes and the stronger the fight or flight response grows. LeDoux, in his 1996 book, *The Emotional Brain: The Mysterious Underpinnings of Emotional Response*, explains it this way: "The brain enters into a vicious cycle of emotional and cognitive excitement and, like a runaway train, just keeps picking up speed."

Erel Shvil, a clinical psychologist and a fellow at Columbia University Medical Center's Trauma and PTSD Program, where he investigates the brain mechanisms of PTSD, says that PTSD is essentially a fear disorder. Those with PTSD reexperience the traumatic event over and over. They often try to avoid the stimuli linked to the event, such as avoiding loud sounds or situations that are not easily assessed and controllable. (Some combat veterans call Walmart "Traumamart" because the store is so large and chaotic.) Those with PTSD are hyper vigilant, always on high alert for the slightest perceived threat.

Those and other symptoms relate directly to how the brain functions during a traumatic event. In the thick of a life-threatening event the brain is in a state of high alert. And in those with PTSD, that state of high alert is easily triggered. Traumatic memories flood back, brought on by things that may seem only peripherally related to the event, forcing people to relive the trauma over and over. They don't sleep well, and they overreact to even the slightest threat because their systems are still responding to a trauma that is months or even years old. The amygdala is overactive, while the parts of the brain that should be overriding the amygdala's red alert—the hippocampus and the frontal cortex—are not doing their jobs. Severe stress has even been shown to shrink parts of the hippocampus and prolonged stress can permanently impair it. While normal memories dissipate over time, traumatic memories can become amplified, and the events that trigger them can change and even broaden, working in the reverse of our usual process.

As Cleland writes in his memoir, *Heart of a Patriot: How I Found the Courage to Survive Vietnam, Walter Reed and Karl Rove*, his memory of the event that maimed him still haunts him decades later:

> *In my mind I replayed the grenade explosion again and again. Ducking under the wash from the chopper blades. Bending over, reaching out. Then, boom! No matter how many times the moment has come flooding back to me, it always ends the same way, always in utter catastrophe. The memory is still there today, buried deep inside the ancient reptile part of my brain. It haunts me in life, always there, always threatening to leap*

back into my consciousness. When it finds me again—sometimes in dark
quiet moments, sometimes at moments of great stress—I am right back
there again on that hill, dying.

Shvil says that those with PTSD have a hard time differentiating between things that should trigger a fear response and things that should not. If, say, a soldier was wounded in an explosion and one of the things he remembers from the explosion was fire, then fire—any fire—could trigger that memory to come flooding back. But these memories, full of dense information and thick with emotion, are much stronger than normal memories. They don't just bring up the memory of terror; they create real terror, as real as if the person were in the thick of the event. As Cleland says, even decades later the memory puts him right back in that place again, flooded with fear and helplessness, fighting for his life.

These problems, it turns out, are not just restricted to memories of the traumatic event. Shvil replicated a well-known Harvard experiment for his own research that found that people with PTSD continue to have a hard time separating other, unrelated, threatening stimuli from innocuous ones. For his version of the experiment, Shvil worked with thirty-one people with PTSD and twenty-five trauma-exposed people without the disorder. He hooked them up to a functional magnetic resonance imaging machine that measures activity in different areas of the brain and a sweat sensor that measures fear and other stress responses, and he showed both groups an image of an office. In that office was a lamp. When the lamp flashed yellow, nothing happened. When it flashed blue, the participants were shocked 60 percent of the time, creating an association between the blue light and pain—training the subjects to fear the blue light. Then he changed the background to that of a library and showed the subjects blue and yellow light without any shock at all. The goal was to override the association between the blue light and the shock with new information—that they would not be shocked in the library.

The participants returned twenty-four hours later. This time he showed them the library—the safe environment—and the flashing light. By measuring sweat and brain activity, he was able to tell that those without PTSD were unconcerned that they would be shocked again—they had learned and remembered from the previous day that in this environment the light did not indicate a shock was coming. They picked up on the meaning of the clues in their environment before their fear response was triggered. The amygdala, the brain's alarm bell, was being overridden by other parts of the brain, as it should be.

But those with PTSD reacted differently. When the lamp flashed blue they began to sweat and indicated that they were fearful that they would be shocked, even in the library—the safe environment. The amygdala was running wild on its own. The hippocampus, the part of the brain that helps with understanding context, was not working in the same way for them as it was for those who did not have PTSD. They were unable to erase the previous fear memory—that the blue light was likely to shock them in the office environment—with the new information, that the blue light would not shock them in the new library environment. Their brains were not picking up on the importance of the context, just like their brains were not picking up on the environmental queues related to the memories of their traumatic event. Those were the findings of the original Harvard experiment, too. When he replicated the study, Shvil discovered something else. Women and men reacted differently. Women with PTSD were more likely than men to be able to see the contextual cues, but they still did not perform as well as those who were not diagnosed with PTSD. "With PTSD you overgeneralize fear, you see different things as being the same, you miss the crucial differences," says Shvil.

Today PTSD is often treated with cognitive behavioral therapy, which gives survivors tools to manage their distress and can involve talking through their experiences over and over again to try to desensitize them to the experience and to extinguish the fearful associations with the event. The memory never goes away, but over time (and with repeated exposure) those suffering from PTSD can begin to break their associations with particular sights, smells, or sounds.

Cleland was able to find a way to manage his anger and bitterness. He says that after struggling with depression and anxiety, he simply decided that he would fight, that he would push forward inch by inch. He knew that he couldn't sit at home in his parents' house for the rest of his life. He had to do something. And he did. At the age of twenty-eight he became the youngest person ever to serve in the Georgia State Senate. "As a veteran overcoming physical disability, it gave me strength," he says. "If I lost the state senate race, what were they going to do to me, send me back to Vietnam? What did I have to lose?" When Jimmy Carter rose from the Georgia governor's mansion to the White House in 1976, he made Cleland the head of the Veterans Administration, a job that Cleland cherished.

"It was so valuable to me that I got a chance to help those who were also suffering," Cleland says. "I had a powerful sense of validation that somehow all the crap has some kind of meaning." In 1996 Cleland won the election for a U.S. Senate seat from Georgia. It was a remarkable accomplishment for anyone, let alone a man who had lost both legs and an arm, who decades before could barely imagine any life for himself at all. Little did Cleland know, the worst was yet to come.

In 2002, Cleland lost his race for reelection. For any politician, losing an election is certainly a hard blow. But it is also part of the job. Yet for Cleland, the loss was catastrophic. "That was far worse than when I came back from Vietnam," Cleland says. "When I got blown up, I had my survival instinct. I fought like hell to survive. But when I lost my election, it was more than just losing, it was the elimination of a life where I had support. I had staff. I had people who helped me out. I had income. I had friends and then boom! I didn't have any of that anymore."

Cleland left the senate feeling that his whole world had been taken from him. All of the supports that he had carefully built up to keep him focused, functioning, and thriving had been pulled away. The only thing that was left was the trauma of Vietnam, which had remained lurking in the background, in the recesses of his brain. "There was a powerful sense of vulnerability, an overwhelming, massive, great depression. Anxiety kicked up, triggering the PTSD I'd kept at bay," he says. In a flash he would once again be lying on the ground beneath those chopper blades bleeding to death. Cleland hit bottom. He would sit at home, consumed with thoughts of death and war. He felt like something horrible was about to happen at any moment and there was nothing he could do to escape it. His mind stopped working. He felt shattered, like he had no hope, no future, that his life was over.

For Cleland, the most traumatic event he experienced was not the obvious trauma: losing his arm and legs to a stray grenade. Instead it was a career derailment: losing his senate seat. That is hardly what one would consider a traumatic event. But for him, it was. Defining trauma by the event that causes it is not an easy thing to do. In fact the definition of trauma has changed every time the American Psychiatric Association publishes a new manual of mental disorders.

When PTSD was first introduced into the *DSM* in 1980, the definition of what kind of trauma could trigger the disorder was rigid: an event outside the range of normal human experience that would cause distress in most people. But over time it has become apparent to many in the field that the trauma in a traumatic event is more closely associated with a person's perception of the event than the event itself. Bereavement is a common cause of the symptoms associated with post-traumatic stress, yet death is a universal human experience.

And being injured in a horrific event is hardly a requirement for a trauma to cause high levels of distress. Following the terrorist attacks of 9/11 in New York City, many residents felt traumatized. But the reality is that very few of those people were physically injured. With rare exceptions, those who were close enough to be physically harmed by the attack did not survive. But for residents of lower Manhattan, those anywhere near the site that day, the friends and relatives of those killed, the emergency workers who lost friends and colleagues and toiled at Ground Zero for months recovering body parts, the post-traumatic stress was widespread. About 20 percent of those who simply happened to live south of Canal Street in lower Manhattan were estimated to have PTSD.

Trauma, or, more accurately, what people perceive as traumatic, is subjective. Everyone perceives an event and its meaning a little differently. What is earth-shattering and traumatic for a rookie cop may be unmoving for a veteran. The same goes for soldiers. Those on their fourth tour in Afghanistan may have acclimated themselves to a level of violence that a soldier on his first deployment would find overwhelming. Or that experienced soldier may suffer even more from the cumulative trauma he has experienced over so many years in a war zone.

Tedeschi and Calhoun, in their work as clinicians, have come to see trauma in just this way. It doesn't matter much what the event is. In order for an event to spur growth, what matters is that it shakes the person to the core, and that can occur in an incredible variety of ways. "We define trauma in terms of its effect on the individual more than a particular event," says Tedeschi. "We think that the subjective appraisal of the impact of the event is going to tell you a lot more about the effect than what kind of event it was."

And so, viewed from this perspective, all sorts of events have the potential to be traumatic—even, in some cases, things that happen to someone else. Post-traumatic stress and post-traumatic growth have been recorded in the spouses of cancer survivors, a kind of vicarious trauma and growth. People can be traumatized by even the happiest of situations: childbirth. One study found that nearly 9 percent of women exhibited the symptoms of full-blown PTSD following childbirth, and that 18 percent exhibited some of the symptoms. Another study found that more than half of the women surveyed after childbirth experienced some level of post-traumatic growth. Though we generally don't think of something as common and usually happy as childbirth as potentially traumatic, for some it certainly can be, as can many other life events, even severe financial loss.

In 2008, after the news broke about Bernard Madoff's $65 billion Ponzi scheme, Audrey Freshman, a clinical therapist in Rockville Centre on Long Island, set up a support group for Madoff's victims. More and more people began reaching out to tell their stories and seek support. Many of them were elderly, and a large number of them had lost their entire life savings at a time when they were nearing retirement. Moreover, in many cases the government came after these people to try to retrieve any funds that they had withdrawn over time, to be used to pay back other victims. They lost everything and the loss was front-page news. Many commentators wondered how the victims could have been unaware of the crooked nature of Madoff's scheme. The victims were embarrassed, and they found little sympathy for their plight.

Freshman was surprised to find that there was no research on the traumatic effects of catastrophic financial loss—after all, everyone had heard of bankers throwing themselves out of windows after the stock market crash of 1929. She decided to study the Madoff victims. Nine months after Madoff was arrested, she surveyed 170 victims using standard screenings for PTSD and other factors like depression and alcohol and drug use. She found that a shockingly high 55.7 percent of those she surveyed met the criteria for PTSD. "Some of these people lost everything, they lost the ability to pay for themselves in old age, they lost their freedom and sense of well-being and faith in the American government," says Freshman. "They felt like they failed. They were humiliated and shamed."

After more than a year of misery, Max Cleland began working with a therapist at Walter Reed. Sometimes he would just sit in her office and cry. He realized that he had never healed from his PTSD. Instead it had festered inside, covered over by his accomplishments and the support system he had built in elected office. Losing his job ripped that support away and the horrible wounds were opened up again. But over the course of two years, with group therapy and medication to help him manage his symptoms, he learned to gain some control over his PTSD and start on the path to finding new meaning in his life.

Cleland has suffered greatly over the course of his life. But he also changed dramatically, finding inner strength, meaningful work, close relationships. The depths of his reactions to his trauma have helped to spur his changes. But the relationship between the severity of the trauma and level of growth is not always straightforward.

Many studies have found that those with less severe trauma report less growth. But they also found that those with the most severe traumatic experiences (as measured by the individual's assessment of their impact or in some cases the severity of their PTSD) also report lower levels of growth. What researchers wind up with is an inverted U-shaped graph. Those reporting a midrange of trauma (the bump in the inverted U) report the most growth. Those at either end report the least growth.

Tedeschi says that for those at the far end of the spectrum, survivors of genocide, for example, their world may be so shattered, the trauma so all encompassing, that they may have little left with which to rebuild. They may become functional, but significant growth may be unlikely. And those who experience only a mild traumatic experience may not have their world and sense of self disturbed enough to force them through the process required for change to occur.

It is the midrange of experience where most studies show the greatest potential for growth. That midrange is quite broad, encompassing those who suffer from full-blown PTSD and those who manifest only some post-traumatic stress symptoms. It even can include those who didn't directly suffer the trauma but are close to those who did. One study, conducted on the spouses of former Israeli prisoners of war by Rachel Dekel, a professor at the Bar-Ilan University School of Social Work in Israel, found that the more severe the level of PTSD experienced by the soldier, the higher the level of distress and the higher the level of growth that the spouse experienced. "The couple felt like, 'we did it, we stayed together,' the joint struggle over-coming difficulties, the struggle, the journey gave it all some mean-ing," she says.

Among those at the opposite end of the scale, those who suffer the most, PTSD is no impediment to growth. In fact, Tedeschi says, PTSD often sets the stage for the kind of suffering and reassessment that is often required for growth. When a person is suffering from the symptoms of PTSD, that is the point at which he is beginning to try to make sense of the trauma, integrating his experience back into his everyday life and trying to rebuild his sense of self. Once the person is able to have some level of control over the fear that is part of the experience of PTSD, he can begin the process of making meaning of his experiences. It is only those who have experienced the most extreme forms of trauma and those who suffer the highest levels of PTSD who may find that they cannot respond in some positive way from the event.

Yet there are outliers. And a few studies do challenge the idea that those who suffer the most trauma, those with the most severe PTSD, grow less or not at all. A study published in 2012 by researchers in Is-rael surveyed former prisoners of war there three times over seventeen years, asking about their stress reactions to their experience and about their growth. The researchers found that the greater the PTSD soldiers reported in 1991, the greater the growth they reported in 2003. Simi-larly, the greater the PTSD reported in 2003, the greater the levels of growth reported in 2008. "We found that over time, PTSD was not just correlated with growth, but that it predicted growth," says the study's lead author, Sharon Dekel, an instructor of psychology at Harvard Medical School (no relation to Rachel Dekel of Bar-Ilan University, mentioned earlier). Her findings mirror those by William Sledge published three decades earlier. Sledge's study of American airmen held by the North Vietnamese similarly found that the longer the soldiers were held captive, and the worse they were treated, the more positive change they reported. For some people, it seems, the more they suffer, the more they grow.

Today Cleland is the secretary of the American Battle Monuments Commission, and he says his life is good. He exercises and focuses on his spiritual and psychological recovery every day. Cleland, who is an only child, had always been fiercely independent. But he has learned that he needs others and he values his friends in a new way. "Knowing that I need other people is growth," says Cleland. "I know that I cannot do this by myself." He has been able to look back at his life and acknowledge his own strength and appreciate the meaning that he has been able to find in his life's work. "I am reasonably happy. I am still a human being. I have injuries. I live with them every second; it will never escape me. I have to deal with that. It triggers powerful emotions, stuff you can't even imagine," he says. At the same time, he says, "I thank God for my little job now. I am thankful for my friends and my ability to enjoy the day and thrive. I am grateful. I can't believe how good my life is."

Cleland's life, his injuries and scars, physical and psychological, are complex. The horror and terror of that explosion, the life-altering moment, are indelibly mixed with his achievements, survival, a life of service that he is proud of, meaningful goals achieved, and ongoing mental and physical challenges. That complex and often contradictory trajectory, which refuses to adhere to any neat chronological progression, may actually be the most accurate way to think about trauma and growth and post-traumatic stress. Rachel Yehuda, the director of the Traumatic Stress Studies Division at the Mount Sinai School of Medicine says that for a long time researchers and clinicians thought that the body and mind were stressed by trauma and that after a certain period of time they just went back to normal. They thought so in part because that is how the physiology of trauma was perceived. The most common marker of trauma, adrenaline, which the body releases in stressful situations, quickly dissipates.

"We kept expecting people to go back to normal because their biology does," says Yehuda. Then psychologists began looking at PTSD in terms of illness, using a model that says that some people get sick and some people do not. But perhaps that is not quite right, either. We are starting to learn that contrary to what we once thought, biology does not always go back to normal. Shvil's experiment with the blinking lights shows that the brains of those with PTSD do work differently than those without the disorder, sometimes for long periods after the trauma occurs. One researcher has found that the brains of those with PTSD are different enough from others that brain images can be used as a diagnostic tool for PTSD with about 90 percent accuracy. Ki Goosens's experiments with rats show one hormone the body releases in stressful situations remains elevated for very long periods, which may also be driving changes in the brain that remain over time.

Today we are gaining a profoundly different way of understanding what it means to survive a traumatic experience. "Trauma causes change. There are a lot of opinions out there about how that change manifests, but you just don't stay the same. That is a really radical idea," says Yehuda. "You do recover in some ways, but that recovery doesn't actually involve returning to the baseline. It involves recalibration towards something new, and PTSD is a way of describing that in a very negative light, and post-traumatic growth is a way of describing that in a very positive light."

Not everyone grows from trauma, but for most of us, the opportunity is there. And researchers have spent decades learning about who is most likely to grow and what kinds of activities and circumstances are most likely to foster post-traumatic growth.

PART TWO

The Essential Tools for Growth

The Six Keys to Transforming Trauma into Positive Change

CHAPTER 4

Telling a New Story

Why Your Narrative Makes or Breaks Growth

OUTSIDE OF GALWAY TECHNICAL INSTITUTE, IN WESTERN IRELAND, a group of students ate lunch on the curb of a grassy traffic circle in the center of the school's parking lot on a spring afternoon. The college is contained in a single, aging building about the size of a large high school and the island of green in the parking lot is the closest thing it's got to a college quad. Nearby, a few others stood by the building's front door smoking beneath a sign that asks students not to smoke in the doorway. Everyone was dressed in baggy pants, T-shirts, and hoodies, except for Shane Mullins. He wore a dark blue suit and a faintly pink shirt unbuttoned at the collar. His red hair was cut short and styled rigidly with gel. Mullins walked briskly past the lounging students without pause or much notice. Though his right leg moved much more slowly and stiffly than the left, leaving him with a pronounced limp, he appeared driven, focused, in a hurry to get where he was going as he passed the smokers in the doorway on his way inside.

Just a few years ago, Mullins was one of those students—an unlikely turn of events given that he'd left high school at age sixteen.

Today he was arriving to give a presentation, to tell the surprising story of his life and how it changed after a terrible accident.

After he dropped out of school, Mullins began working for his father as a block layer, building homes in the frenzy of the Irish housing boom. He also worked on the family farm in the rural town of Monivea, where he grew up. "He was a typical teenager," says his mother, Rose Mullins. He played rugby and soccer and spent time with his friends. And, like many Irish teens, he spent a lot of time at the pub. "I was a wild young fellow and I was always fighting," says Mullins. But that never stopped him from working hard, too. "I was a good worker, I had the farm. I wasn't really thinking about life. I was just thinking about money for the week," says Mullins. By the time he was seventeen and a half years old, Mullins had saved up enough to buy a car.

About six month later, Mullins was having one of those wild nights. He and a friend had started drinking in the afternoon. They went to a party. They wound up at a pub where they drank until they were thrown out. Then they got into Mullins's car. He managed to drive a few hundred yards before he ran off the road. The car rolled over. As it came down on the roof, a stone pillar crashed through the top of the car and into Mullins's head, leaving him unconscious. By the time he got to the hospital, he was in a coma. His situation looked so bleak that doctors told his parents to consider donating his organs.

Four days later Mullins awoke. He jokes that his head swelled up like E.T.'s because of all the bleeding in his brain. He lost the sight in his left eye. His right side was nearly paralyzed; he could barely move his leg or his arm. He developed a terrible MRSA infection. He was on a feeding tube for three months. The whole time his family rarely left his side. When he was wheeled out of the hospital three months later on his way to Dublin for rehabilitation, he weighed just ninety-eight pounds.

As severe as those injuries were, the most debilitating injury Mullins suffered was to his brain. Traumatic brain injuries have become the signature wound of the Iraq and Afghanistan wars—often the result of the concussive blasts from roadside bombs. But brain injuries also affect many civilians, especially those who survive violent car crashes. Each injury is different. Some heal with time and effort; others will never get better, leaving their victims struggling with a host of problems, from impaired speech and movement to memory disorders and problems with decision making, impulse control, and even cognitive ability.

When that stone pillar crashed through the roof of his car that night, it damaged Mullins's cerebellum, the part of the brain that, among other things, aids in balance and coordination as well as language skills. Mullins was confined to a wheelchair, in part because he was having trouble moving his right leg, but also because he had almost no sense of balance and fell over as soon as he tried to stand up. When he opened his mouth to speak he'd say different words than he intended. Often he just cursed, and it seemed that it was always at the worst possible time. He could never predict what was going to come out of his mouth.

After months of strength training in Dublin, he learned to walk again, but with a crutch to help with his balance. With time, practice, and therapy his speech improved as well. As soon as he got home, feeling that he was well on the road to recovery, he did what just about anyone would do: he tried to take up his old life again. He started going out to the pub with friends. "They used to call me the wiggly-wobbly wonder," says Mullins. "I'd wiggle in, I'd wobble out, and then wonder how I was going to get home." He quickly discovered that his brain injury did not mix well with alcohol. "I was drunk after one pint. My cerebellum was damaged and my balance just went," he says. "I couldn't walk after two. I couldn't even go to the bathroom. I would drink myself silly. I was drinking away the pain that I was in."

His old friends, everyone he knew in his very small, close-knit town, looked at him with pity. Because he couldn't walk straight and often couldn't say what he meant, people treated him like he was mentally disabled, which made him angry. His family, which had been a remarkable source of support, was getting fed up with having to haul him home from the pub and take care of him. More than once Mullins contemplated suicide. "Most things depressed me and got me down and that would make me drink," he says.

He knew that he had to do something. Despite his desire to take up his old life again, it was clear that he could not. He had to change, to find a new direction that was compatible with the unforgiving limitations of his brain injury. The first step, he knew, was to stop drinking. So he went back to Dublin to an inpatient facility specializing in brain injuries.

It was not easy. He was bitter and angry. He felt it was unfair that he had to quit drinking while everyone else went about their lives—and their drinking—without any of the struggles he faced. But Mullins stuck with it and was soon sober. While he was in Dublin, he started taking classes to learn more about his brain injury. And he was required to see a therapist, something he dreaded and avoided. He didn't think that he needed help. And, in truth, he was afraid. He'd never talked openly to anyone about his feelings. The first time Mullins went, he didn't say anything. Instead he just let the therapist talk. But soon he found himself opening up, sometimes taking up more than his allotted hour. "I learned that it was doing me so much good, it was just unbelievable," he says. "It has helped me so much in life."

While he was getting sober and going through therapy, Mullins decided that he needed to make a big change. He finally accepted the hard truth—that he could not have his old life back. But perhaps he could find a way to begin on the path to a different life. Mullins told his mother that he wanted to go to college. "She started laughing at me and I started laughing as well; it was hard to imagine," he says. Nonetheless, the high school dropout decided to give it a try. He started at Galway Technical Institute in 2010. Despite his deep motivation, he found the work overwhelming. Just as he thought he had failed again and considered dropping out, he had the luck of meeting two influential teachers. One of them convinced him to cut down his course load and focus on just two classes so he'd be more likely to succeed. The other taught a communications class.

Over the years since his accident, Mullins had been thinking about his healing, his therapy and sobriety, taking notes on what was working and what wasn't. He came up with a system that he calls D'MESS—the core principles that he says were instrumental in helping him confront and overcome all that he's faced since the accident. D'MESS is an acronym standing for Determination, Motivation, Emotional Support, and Social Life. That communications teacher, Mary McGuinness, eventually helped Mullins put together a PowerPoint presentation detailing the accident and its aftermath, how he became sober and began pursuing a new life and how this system helped him. Since leaving the school, Mullins has given the presentation to youth groups, schools, and other organizations all over Ireland. He's been on TV and radio shows. He's been written up in the paper. The BBC did a radio documentary about him.

At Galway Technical Institute, Mullins gave his presentation to the same communications class where he developed the talk. About two dozen students, both teachers, and his mother and sister looked on as he spoke. He told his story, showing pictures of himself in the hospital, in a wheelchair, drunk in a pub. He talked openly about his struggles with sobriety and the times he was held in mental hospitals because of his suicidal impulses. He discussed it all with great humor, touching on binge drinking, mental health, life choices, determination, and character—all without being preachy or condescending. He told them, "It was my idea to go to college. I took initiative with my own life. Was it hard? Absolutely. But I kept on going. I kept doing it. I found new hobbies and interests. Now I am all over the country. I've been on TV and radio programs. These are really good things." Mullins said that he hoped his accomplishments can help others: "I hope that I can inspire and motivate you. Everyone needs a little help in life."

During his talk, it became clear that he was doing something else, too. He was going through an elaborate and very public process of explaining how he became the new person he is today. He understands that he can never be the person he was before he ran his car into that stone pillar. That person is gone as surely as if he died that day, and he has been forced to reinvent himself. These presentations are one way of reintroducing himself to the world.

Such a severe accident, the kind that leaves one with lifelong struggles, is not supposed to change a person in such a positive way. Drunk driving accidents should not transform a high school dropout and a block layer to a person who puts on suits and makes presentations. But that is Mullins's story. And the presentation is his way of explaining it to anyone who will listen. "If I hadn't had my accident, I would not have gone through these changes, not one of them," he said before his talk. "I respect people more. Everyone seems to fight their own battles. And I have a lot more fight and determination. I'm very happy with the new person that I have become. My interests in life have totally changed and I've found the right road. I'm working towards my goals and that feels good."

Not everything is perfect, of course. Mullins gets frustrated with his family and the people in his small town who, he says, don't understand who he has become. Because of his brain injury—the issues with balance and fatigue, his blindness in one eye—he has not been able to work, even around the farm, where a wobble at the wrong time can lead to serious injury. And Mullins says that his father, whom he once worked with side by side, has a hard time understanding both the limitations of his injuries and his changes. "Of course I get angry sometimes. Of course I get frustrated," says Mullins. "But I'm on the right road." It's a road that he hopes will lead to a career as a presenter on a radio or TV program, a high bar, he understands, but just like in rehab, he says it is about taking small steps in the right direction. "I am rebuilding myself as a whole new person," he says.

Creating a New Narrative

Mullins had to reinvent himself, come up with an entirely new story about who he was, what he expected from life, and how he could achieve that new vision. The accident and resulting brain injury was the catalyst, the thing that pushed him to abandon his old self and to embrace someone new. He had to find a new narrative. The stories people tell about who they are and what their lives can and can't be are remarkably important. They can trap individuals in a life that no longer works or can open the door to something new and transformative. Traumatic events have the capacity not only to upend those stories, but they can also be the catalyst that forces people to find new and often better narratives for ourselves.

Ronnie Janoff-Bulman, a professor at the University of Massachusetts at Amherst who studied trauma and change for more than a decade, theorized that particularly in Western culture, people develop firmly held beliefs that are incompatible with traumatic experience. They believe that the world is benevolent, that the world is meaningful and just, and that we are good people. In this worldview, bad things don't happen to good people—especially to oneself. And while people understand intellectually that terrible things can happen to anyone at any time, each of us also, quite irrationally, believes that those things are unlikely to happen to us.

This concept is so well understood that researchers have given it a name: unrealistic optimism. And they have been studying it for decades. In one striking study published in 1996, three British researchers went to a bungee-jumping site to learn how people perceived risk. They asked first-time bungee jumpers whether they would be more or less likely than a "typical" jumper to be injured in the 160-foot free fall and ensuing high-velocity bounces. Then they posed the same question to the friends and family members assembled to watch the leap. The friends and family members said the obvious and rational thing—the risks to their loved ones were the same as they were to a "typical" jumper.

But the bungee jumpers had a very different response. They overwhelmingly said that a "typical" jumper was more likely to be injured than they were. That answer makes no sense. Obviously the risk is the same. But perhaps that attitude is what helped to convince them to go bungee jumping in the first place.

This way of looking at the world extends far beyond plunging off a platform. People have the same misguided way of thinking about illness, natural disasters, and other calamities. It's one of the reasons why Californians don't fret about earthquakes. In part it's why, despite auto accidents and pedestrian fatalities and terrorist attacks, people still get up and go outside and live their lives. Everyone knows that these events happen, but no one can get through life thinking that calamity lies around every corner.

According to Janoff-Bulman, people develop a core sense of themselves based on the moral universe they think they live in. She calls it the assumptive self—the individual's idea of themselves as good, of living in a safe world, of being rewarded for being a decent person. It's an idea that Tedeschi and Calhoun, the researchers who pioneered the study of post-traumatic growth, adopted early on to explain how trauma can change identity. When bad things happen to someone good, it tears down that assumptive self. And much of the psychological anguish that people confront has to do with the loss of this worldview and the identity that they carried with them their entire lives. In this way of looking at the world, when someone does get cancer or loses a loved one in an earthquake or is gravely injured in a bungee-jumping accident, asking "Why me?" is not only a legitimate question, but one that demands to be answered.

That question can be a dead end—there is no good answer to it. But for some, understanding that they cannot answer that question can set them on the path to overturning their old assumptive self. It's a journey that can be very painful. Part of the struggle of post-traumatic stress, Calhoun and Tedeschi have found, is derived from the inconsistency between the old assumptive self and the new reality imposed by the traumatic event. Trauma upends our entire understanding of the world we live in, how it works, and our own place in it.

The ability to abandon the old assumptive self or narrative and to develop a new one is at the heart of the process that can result in post-traumatic growth, says the University of Nottingham's Stephen Joseph. "People are always telling themselves stories; it is how we make sense of the significance of what has happened to us," he says. "In the wake of trauma, people are often telling themselves stories of mental defeat and hopelessness. And they need to be in a position to begin reframing their story, as one that looks to the future and begins to view things in a beneficial way."

To do that, people need to be able to integrate the new traumatic experience into their lives. According to theories advanced by developmental psychologist Jean Piaget, we usually assimilate new information by fitting the new experience into our existing way of understanding the world, which keeps that worldview intact. Joseph uses the example of a child playing with blocks who is handed a magnet. When she *assimilates* the magnet, she stacks it on top of her tower as if it were another block—the magnet is being absorbed into her worldview of objects as blocks.

But if the child discovers that the magnet attracts metal and begins playing with the object as a magnet, then she is *accommodating* the new information—building a new construct that takes into account the different properties of this new object. Similarly, survivors must reconstruct their worldview into one that accommodates the new properties embodied by the trauma. If they don't, they will be constantly pushing back against the memories and associations of the event and all they lost with anger and frustration. They will continue to try (and fail) to build the tower higher using the magnet as a block. But if they do manage to accommodate the traumatic experience by understanding that it requires a new worldview, the trauma can become part of the foundation for a new way of understanding themselves, perhaps even the starting point for a whole new and better life. Magnets, after all, can do many things that blocks cannot.

Shane Mullins was in just such a situation. Initially he acted as if the accident didn't affect him, that he had no need to change, that he could just pick up his old life where he left off. But the realities of his injury wouldn't let him. He was pushed by the pain and frustration of all he survived to the point where he could see that drinking was inhibiting him. And once he was sober, he clearly understood that he had to find a new direction for his life. His old life was gone, and he could see that he now had an opportunity to create a new one. By accommodating what had occurred—the accident, the brain injury, his changes and limitations—he was pushed to find a new direction, new goals, a whole new way of understanding who he could be.

One of the most important things that helped Mullins drive toward that change—to see that it was possible and to inspire himself to rethink his life—was, oddly, a blockbuster film. Before his accident he'd seen the 1995 historical epic *Braveheart*, about William Wallace, who in the late thirteenth century led the Scottish in an uprising against the English. The film had never meant much to him, but after the accident he became obsessed with the movie.

In the film, directed by and starring Mel Gibson, Wallace's life is portrayed as a series of traumatic events that propel him into ever more important roles. When Wallace was just a child, his father and brother were killed by the English and he fled the country. He returned to Scotland as an adult and married his childhood friend, only to see her captured and executed by English troops. Wallace responded by attacking the nearby occupying garrison and defeating them. With Wallace leading them, the Scots rose up, defeating English troops, taking several cities and even invading England. Wallace was eventually betrayed by his countrymen and handed over to the English. He was offered a quick death if he would only utter the word *mercy* but he refused. Though in the most horrible pain, he wouldn't take the English offer; instead he shouted "Freedom!" in defiance of his torturers before he died.

After Mullins's accident, whenever he felt down or overwhelmed, he'd put the movie on. "When he was feeling low, *Braveheart* used to boost him up again," says his mother, Rose. "He got a lot of inspiration from that movie."

And he still watches the movie to this day. "The *Braveheart* speech, I'll have it on this evening," he said before his talk in Galway. "My determination and motivation especially came from William Wallace. Each time things got hard for him, he saw through things and fought even harder and that's what I did. Each time things got hard for me, I thought about him and I went on fighting a bit harder."

The film and the story of Wallace's life provided a map for Mullins, a role model to follow, someone who showed him that anything can be overcome by determination, and that trauma can be turned on its head to provide a springboard for something better.

"The presence of a role model is important for growth," says Calhoun. Several studies have shown this to be true. One, by LIU Post assistant professor Tzipi Weiss, who studied growth across dozens of cultures, examined seventy-two breast cancer survivors. Some of those cancer survivors had contact with another survivor who reported growth. Weiss found that just having contact with someone who had grown was one of the biggest factors in predicting posttraumatic growth. In addition, those women who knew someone who had grown reported higher levels of positive change than did other survivors.

Weiss knows firsthand just how much role models can help. In 1995 she fell ill, likely as a result of exposure to toxic chemicals. She was so sick that at times she could not leave her bed and was in severe pain. Traditional medicine offered no help. A nurse suggested that she start recording even the tiniest moments of positive feeling. She noticed how just watching her children or her husband made her happy. She read Viktor Frankl's *Man's Search for Meaning*. And she found someone else who had survived a terrible illness, whose story acted as a model for her. Eventually she was diagnosed with and treated for liver toxicity and her health improved. Now, she says, she is closer to her family and friends, appreciates her life in a way she hadn't before, and sees herself as stronger and more capable.

For Weiss, having a role model was crucial. "It doesn't even have to be a specific person's story of recovery," she says. "It could be a work of art, a metaphor, a fairy tale or myth, even an element of nature. What is important is that you see the possibility of benefiting from suffering. Once you have that concept, you are more likely to start looking for it."

Mullins knew the *Braveheart* story and found that after his accident, he could use its uplifting message to his advantage. "When Wallace said he was going to invade England on their own turf, they [his fellow Scots] all started laughing at him," says Mullins. "He just walked away and went out. Same with me. I want to invade brain injury on its own turf, which I'm doing. They might laugh and I'll walk away. Who has the last laugh? Me."

Time to Reflect

Mullins was able to find a new narrative for himself. But how? What was the process that led him there and helps others to define themselves anew after trauma?

After a traumatic experience it's common to think about the event, even to the point of obsession. Survivors often suffer from intrusive thoughts—images of the event that come back to them with little warning, creating tremendous anxiety. People may try to avoid thinking about the event entirely to forestall these images and memories, and research suggests that may actually be a healthy and necessary part of recovery, but only for a time.

If the process stops there, this kind of avoidance can ultimately impede healing and growth. Images of the event will continue to plague the survivor, regardless of his or her efforts to avoid the triggers that bring them flooding in. And choosing to wallow in negative emotions for too long can become debilitating and an impediment to change. What is required instead is something Tedeschi and Calhoun call deliberate rumination.

Deliberate rumination is a different kind of thought process, one driven by the individual, not the trauma. It is not wallowing or obsessing. When someone is deliberately ruminating on a problem, he is actively involved in thinking about how the event has impacted him, what it means for him, and how he can live his life going forward given the challenges that the event has posed. When deliberately ruminating, the trauma survivor is actively tackling the challenges that the trauma has introduced to the assumptive world. Deliberate rumination is the way that people begin to rebuild themselves.

For a paper published in 2013, Suzanne Danhauer, an associate professor of social sciences and health policy at Wake Forest School of Medicine, paired up with Tedeschi and Calhoun to study growth in patients with acute leukemia. Those with the disease are often admitted immediately upon diagnosis and face long hospital stays and powerful chemotherapy treatments. They can acquire severe infections because of their low white blood cell counts. The chemotherapy can result in sores in their mouths and gastrointestinal tracts, hair loss, nausea, weight loss, and fatigue. Patients undergoing treatment for acute leukemia can suffer from depression, anxiety about the illness coming back, and sleep loss. The researchers wanted to find out whether these patients reported growth and, among those who did, whether they went through the process of deliberate rumination that Tedeschi and Calhoun had outlined.

Danhauer, Tedeschi, and Calhoun measured how much these sixty-six leukemia patients deliberately ruminated on their problems versus how much they were plagued by intrusive thoughts. What they found, even among this group right after diagnosis and during treatment, confirmed the central place that deliberate rumination holds in the growth process. Generally post-traumatic growth increased over each of the time periods while distress fell—the further along patients were in chemotherapy, the more growth and the less distress they reported. They also found strong correlations between the challenges to core beliefs—how much these individuals' assumptive worlds had been shattered by the diagnosis—and growth. And they found a positive correlation between deliberate rumination and growth.

Those who reported growth recognized that leukemia and their struggle with it had changed how they looked at the world for the better. Their inclination to think about the disease, mull it over, and consider the future was the key element that helped them to experience growth. "It is not the actual trauma that is causing the change," says Danhauer. "It is how people interpret what happens, how what they believe about themselves and life and the world gets shaken up, not the trauma itself that forces people to experience growth."

Something like a leukemia diagnosis and treatment or a serious physical injury also affords people long stretches of time during which they have little to do other than lie in a hospital bed and heal or undergo treatment. They may be in a lot of pain and facing severe physical and psychological struggle, but they also wind up with a lot of time on their hands. That can help them begin that deliberate ruminative process.

George Nickel was given such a break, one that forced him to reconsider his life, to reinvent himself anew, but it didn't take place in a hospital bed.

Nickel joined the army right after he graduated from high school in Youngstown, Ohio, in 1989. He served for eight years, until he couldn't take the constant moving from military town to military town anymore. He left the army in 1997 and moved to Boise, Idaho, where he worked as a prison guard. In 2006 a friend told him that his reserve unit was shipping out to Iraq. Nickel, then thirty-five years old, decided to join up again. After six months of training, he was sent to Iraq as part of a team sweeping roads for improvised explosive devices, or IEDs, and disposing of them. It was nerve-racking and risky work, but also gratifying. "For every bomb we found, that meant that another convoy, another unit was not getting hit," Nickel says. "It was a direct payoff."

Nickel would usually ride in the lead vehicle, often at night when the roads were empty, making patrolling easier but visibility worse. He would scan the road for disturbed dirt or pavement, signs that something had recently been buried. The vehicles sent out signals that jammed wireless communications to stop insurgents from triggering the bombs with cell phones. If his team found something, they would use what he calls a buffalo arm, an appendage on the truck that looks like a backhoe arm with a tined end like a fork, to dig the explosives out of the ground. Once the IED was removed, it was detonated.

Of course, his unit didn't always find the IEDs before their heavily armored trucks rolled over them and were rocked by blasts. The trucks themselves were well protected, he says, but the concussion of the blasts would leave soldiers with back injuries and broken bones. Some were left with harder-to-define problems associated with brain injuries, something that none of them were aware of at the time. "It's like getting hit in the chest but all over at once," says Nickel. "It picks you up and throws you from side to side; you're being tossed around inside a metal can."

In February 2007, insurgents shot down a helicopter north of Fallujah. The bodies were recovered shortly after the crash. Nickel's unit was sent out the next day to clear the road so the helicopter could be recovered, too. The road to the crash site was a prime target, since it was clear that soldiers would be headed that way. Nickel's truck rounded a bend and ran over a massive explosive buried under the pavement. The truck was thrown into the air. The gunner and team leader died instantly. The driver died in the medevac chopper.

Nickel woke in Walter Reed Army Medical Center. He'd lost ten days of memory. He also suffered a broken leg, two broken ribs, a broken scapula, a broken cheekbone, a collapsed lung, and a so-called moderate brain injury. The medical team focused on getting him walking again and healing from his broken bones. However, they offered no treatment for his brain injury, even though his short-term memory problems were obvious. He'd wheel his chair around the hospital in search of appointments that he couldn't find, and often forget about what he was doing in the middle of an activity. After one session with a psychologist he was given some tranquilizers and Zoloft, and he returned to Boise.

Back home Nickel often drove around town unable to recall where he was going or why he'd gotten in the car in the first place. The blast had caused shearing in his prefrontal cortex, the part of the brain that is associated with decision making and other higher functions. To this day he continues to struggle with deficits. "I can't make decisions about anything," he says. "I can look at options in front of me for a few hours and not make a choice." Luckily he began physical therapy in a facility that offered some services for brain injury, mostly for survivors of automobile accidents. Some of his brain functions have improved thanks to therapy. After six months the army released him from its medical hold. Nickel tried to sign up for combat duty again. "I was looking for closure. I wanted to finish what I started," he says. But given his injuries and limitations, he was turned down. Nickel saw it as a total rejection. If I'm not combat deployable then I am useless, he thought.

Though he began working as a prison guard again, Nickel never came to terms with the attack in Iraq that killed so many of his fellow soldiers. "I was in denial about losing my guys. I was avoiding dealing with anything. I had anger issues," he says. "I just started getting home from work and drinking until I passed out."

On a July night in 2009, everything came to a head. Nickel's drinking had been escalating for some time. He had gone about three days with almost no sleep and on the third day he drank a case of beer on his own. Then he noticed that his dog was missing. Nickel was convinced that someone in his apartment building had taken his dog. He grabbed his handgun, an AR-15 rifle, and ninety rounds of ammunition. He tried shooting the locks off two of his neighbors' doors. Someone called 911 and within minutes Nickel found himself facing the police. The officers fired twelve rounds at the armed and drunk veteran—they all missed. Nickel surrendered without firing a shot at the police. He was charged with six felonies.

Since Nickel had worked as a prison guard, he was placed in solitary confinement for his own safety, leaving his cell only for an hour a day to exercise. Initially he felt sorry for himself. But in time he got over that. "I really got to be alone with myself, to reflect on what was going on in my life without any distractions," says Nickel. He began to truly reflect on his career and realized that, rather than being a failure who could not be sent back to combat, he had actually accomplished a lot in his military career. He, like Mullins, also began to face up to the limitations of his brain injury, understanding that he would always have problems with memory and decision making and he could not pretend they would go away. And he finally grieved for the men who had died alongside him in Iraq. "This whole process has really helped me to become clearheaded and focused on what I want to do," he says.

As Nickel prepared for trial, he faced two radically different outcomes. Given his military service and service to the state and because no one was injured, he could be let off lightly with time served and probation. At the other extreme he could face fifteen years in prison if he went to trial and was convicted on all charges. While he was in jail, he was amazed to see an outpouring of support from friends, coworkers, and military colleagues. Some wrote letters of support. Others put money in his jail account so he could buy things at the commissary. They created a Facebook page to build support for his case.

In his eight months in solitary confinement, Nickel had nothing to do but think about his life, his past as well as his future. He was using deliberate rumination, taking charge of who he was going to be. "I decided that if I was going to get out, I was going to reinvent myself," says Nickel. He had enjoyed his appointments with the social workers at the Department of Veterans Affairs and the thought of helping other veterans who were struggling like he was appealed to him. "I decided if I could get out of there, if I was given the opportunity to change, I would go back and help other vets before they got to the point where I was."

Nickel got the opportunity. Prosecutors worked out a generous plea agreement placing Nickel on supervised probation. He was also required to participate in substance abuse and inpatient PTSD programs at a nearby VA hospital. Once that was completed he moved into a sober house and started taking classes at Boise State University. He completed his bachelor's degree and started his master's degree in social work. Nickel also works with law enforcement organizations helping veterans from the recent wars who may be having trouble reintegrating into the civilian world.

That is not to say that everything is easy. School is a challenge. He has memory retention problems from his brain injury. He has to put in a lot more time than others to do his course work, but his friends keep pushing him to stay focused. His new career is meaningful, a different world entirely from where he was before he picked up his guns and went looking for his dog. He even talks publicly about what he's been through. "Being open and forthcoming about what happened to me and the problems that I had has helped me to deal with my own issues. Before it was about internalizing and repressing and denying everything. Now I am an open book," he says. "I love it. It has been amazingly rewarding."

Few of us are locked in a cell and forced to think about our traumas and our lives like Nickel was. His case is an extreme example of how isolation (which for some can be mentally damaging on its own) forced him to undertake the introspection that is required for growth. But solitary confinement is hardly required for that sort of deliberate rumination. Robert Neimeyer, a psychology professor at the University of Memphis, studies grief and personal narrative. Neimeyer says that the pain of these experiences becomes the catalyst that forces the introspection. In a way, a person can only be miserable for so long before he tries to find a way out. "The pain can provide the pivot point," Neimeyer says. "People reach a point where they are just trying to find a way to reach beyond the pain and embrace life again."

Pamela Fischer, a psychologist at the Oklahoma City VA Medical Center, spent a dozen years working in the PTSD unit there. She has worked with many patients like Nickel who are feeling hopeless and guilt-ridden over the death of friends in combat. Like so many other veterans, Nickel's guilt stopped him from moving forward in life and kept him trapped in the past. And who he was in the past was incompatible with who he needed to be in Boise. Fischer helps soldiers to get a more clear-eyed view of events, to find some positives to hold on to, and to forgive themselves for any perceived failings, in much the way that Nickel was able to find pride in his military service. Deliberate rumination, reflecting on the event, she says, can allow a trauma survivor to construct a new view of themselves and the world. "Instead of looking back with guilt and self-loathing and criticism, they are often able to understand their behaviors in the context of the trauma, allowing them to move from self-criticism to acceptance."

Deliberate rumination is at the heart of growth. It's an important process that allows trauma survivors to find new narratives for their lives, new ways of understanding their strengths and possibilities, and more meaningful ways to live.

CHAPTER 5

Relying on Others

Community and Support Are Vital for Change

LATE ON THE NIGHT OF DECEMBER 1, 2006, MARIAM DAVIES, A twenty-five-year-old English telemarketer, was on her way to a club with a dozen friends from work—they were out celebrating her birthday. While the group waited for the tube train at the Tooting Broadway station in South London, a work friend she didn't know that well, Gustav Claassens, scooped her up to give her a hug. He spun her around in a circle. Then he lost his balance and fell, holding on tightly to Davies. The pair plummeted down onto the tube tracks just as a train roared into the station.

Davies felt like she had been smacked in the face. "I got punched in the face when I was in primary school, so that was almost the image I had at that moment, like, shit, I've been punched again," she says. Then she was under the train, trying to move closer to the gap between the platform and the train car above her. "Someone was holding my hand and I strongly remember the feeling of, 'I need to get out,'" she says. "I remember people telling me to keep my eyes open and they kept talking to me, trying to keep me conscious. I

remember feeling worried about my coat because it was my favorite."
And then she felt like she was going to die: "I closed my eyes and
recited a prayer that I was taught as a child and then I felt strangely
at peace."

Once Davies and Claassens could both be pulled from under the
train without causing further injury, they were rushed to a nearby
hospital. Shortly afterward Claassens died from his injuries. Davies's
injuries were catastrophic. Her pelvis was cracked in half from top
to bottom, a complex break doctors call an open book fracture. She
broke her left leg in several places and broke a number of ribs, leaving
her with a punctured lung and other internal injuries including nerve
damage on the right side of her body. Doctors were unsure if she
would ever walk again. She was put on a respirator, given morphine,
and put into a coma. The morphine caused bizarre hallucinations.
"I would be on a hospital bed trying to breathe with arms and legs
all over the place, terrified of closing my eyes because if I closed my
eyes, I would die," she says. "One of the worst things I remember was
seeing Gustav walking towards me; his head was all bandaged up and
I was shouting at him, telling him that he was supposed to be my
friend. He was saying, 'I'm sorry. I'm sorry.' It was so vivid."

Davies's parents came to the hospital to see her every day for seven
months. Her mother brought her meals, ensuring that she rarely ate
hospital food. Her ex-boyfriend, John Davies, rushed to the hospital
as soon as he heard the news. The pair had been together for three
years but had broken up a year before the accident. After Davies was
brought out of the coma, she was amazed at the show of support,
particularly from her family. That was unexpected. For the last decade, she'd had little to do with her parents at all.

Davies had a challenging childhood in a sometimes volatile environment. She had a particularly difficult relationship with her young

mother who was only eighteen when Davies was born. By the time Davies was fifteen she left home and though she wanted to continue with her education, she felt that she had no choice but to drop out of school. She soon got caught up in a series of abusive relationships. She drank and experimented with drugs. She moved from job to job with little sense of what she wanted to accomplish. "I was so angry at the world and unrecognizable to the person I am today," she says.

John first met Davies when they were in their early twenties, and even then he could see that she was struggling. "She was trying to find her identity but there were pressures to be a certain way," says John. "There was this one life that she wanted to lead and then there was the family life. It's hard to figure out who you are when you are being pulled in two different directions." Looking back, Davies is less charitable about herself. "From when I was sixteen up to the point where the accident happened, I was just a bit of wreckage. I was having a great time going out and partying and taking drugs, and my head was all over the place," she says. "I was carrying on like a child."

Davies, whose dark eyes are framed by curly black hair, has an engaging intensity about her that makes it easy to believe she was frustrated with a directionless life of partying and dead-end jobs. Though she dropped out of school, she had always been a good student. And she continued to take classes on her own even though she wasn't a full-time student. She knew deep down that she could do more with her life, but she was never certain how to find the right path. "I had big plans of becoming a journalist, so many big ideas, and the fact that I wasn't pursuing any of them bugged me," she says.

She began seeing John in her early twenties, and things began to improve. Finally she found a positive and loving relationship, one that allowed her to begin to process all that she had been through. After so many years of turmoil, she was finally healing. Then, while riding her bike, she was hit by a bus. She broke her elbow, which resulted in multiple surgeries to restore full mobility. She felt depressed and struggled with low self-esteem. She would erupt in emotional outbursts. She broke up with John and left the country to travel, something she thought would help her to find her way. But, in truth, she was just running from her problems. When she returned she was no more directed. "I knew that I needed to make some changes but I didn't know how," she says. "I would pray for something to happen that would force me out of my life."

That something arrived that terrible evening in December. "I remember when I woke in the hospital, having a really powerful sense that this is what I've been waiting for," she says. In the hospital things began to change. She was surrounded by family and friends. She asked John to get back together with her and he agreed. The nurses, who were about her age and treated her more like a friend than a patient, became a source of support. "I didn't feel isolated or alone or ashamed. I felt accepted and loved," she says. "Those are all the key ingredients, and I can't tell you how lucky I feel with the sequence of events and the way that they happened."

Support from Others Is Crucial

Davies was lucky. Research shows that this type of social support is critical for helping people to heal after traumatic events. Shira Maguen, an associate professor at the University of California, San Francisco School of Medicine and a clinician at the San Francisco VA Medical Center, says trauma survivors need support from those they are close to. "The quality of their relationships really helps carry them through the trauma," says Maguen. "So much energy and resources are spent just trying to meet basic needs in the aftermath of trauma;

it is incredibly helpful to have support from those close family and friends."

Social support has been shown time and again to be a key factor in helping people recover from post-traumatic stress symptoms and even PTSD. A study of mothers in New Orleans five years after Hurricane Katrina found that those with strong social support networks had lower levels of post-traumatic stress symptoms. A study of those affected by the terrorist attacks in New York City on September 11, 2001, found that those with low levels of social support were more likely to report symptoms of PTSD. One study of women traumatized by the war in Bosnia found that social support from friends was the key predictor in whether or not the women developed PTSD.

But this kind of support doesn't last forever. And just as much as support can provide people with the platform they need to move forward, its absence can be devastating. Davies thrived in the hospital. It was a kind of protective bubble—a place where she was supported, surrounded by friends and family, and given the time to reflect, to deliberately ruminate on the experience and how she might use it to change. But seven months later, when she was released, her problems escalated. She had to confront her injuries in the real and unforgiving world. She was in a wheelchair. She felt totally dependent on John or her father to get out of the house and get to appointments and physical therapy, even to get the shopping done. "Going from being fiercely independent to becoming dependent, maybe for the rest of my life, I was experiencing all of these emotions. It was hard for me to gracefully accept," she says.

Though the possibility of being dependent worried her, she also felt increasingly alone. There were fewer visits from friends and family. Once she left the hospital, it was like the alarm had turned off, and now everyone was free to return to their normal lives. She felt as if she had been abandoned to figure things out on her own. "I don't know if I had depression, but I definitely struggled. My mom and dad found it difficult to visit regularly to support me because I was far away. It felt similar to when I was fourteen or fifteen and I ran away from home," she says. "I was twenty-five and thought all that stuff had gone away, and it came back again. I knew that I needed to focus quickly."

Davies was released from the hospital in July. By August she had started an online college course on health care. She knew that she needed to get focused on something, and quickly. While she was in the hospital, she had become concerned with the way that the elderly patients there were treated. Many were on their own, with few friends or family members who visited. She thought that going into counseling might be one way she could help them. Perhaps she could start a service linking these older people with volunteers who could visit and keep them company. In September she started a second course, one in a classroom with a live instructor, an introduction to counseling. And after that first counseling class, she knew she had found her calling. It just felt right.

Davies was able to think this way, to direct her life and career toward helping others, only because of the support she had from those she loved. "Before the accident I was convinced that my parents didn't care about me," says Davies. "And then to wake up and be proven completely incorrect, to see that they love me so much, that they were there every day. All the years of carrying so much resentment and going from one job to the next without any focus, and knowing that I hurt them and was not making them proud. Suddenly it became about what to do." Seeing her parents' unconditional love for her, understanding that they felt that way all along, regardless of what she was doing with her life, motivated her to find a way to reinvent herself.

Davies earned her qualification for counseling and today she and a fellow therapist have their own business providing low-cost therapy services in the South London neighborhood where she lives. It's a community with a large population of first- and second-generation immigrants just like Davies—her mother is from India and her father is from Mauritius. Despite her years of psychological turmoil and self-destructive behavior, she'd never considered going to counseling, let alone pursuing it as a career—it just wasn't part of the world she grew up in. By working in this community, she is hoping that more people like her will take advantage of the counseling services she offers. Perhaps she could prevent another person from having to face their problems on their own like she did. Davies also works as a mentor for low-income youth, helping them find a path in life toward a positive and meaningful future.

While Davies's transformation is remarkable and dramatic, it's not surprising that such an outpouring of support helped to get her there. There is a rich body of research tying social support to growth. In 2006 Maguen published a study of combat veterans from the 1990 Persian Gulf War. She found that the single best predictor of post-traumatic growth was the level of social support the soldier had following his or her deployment. A supportive structure of family and friends made growth possible.

Others have found similar results with cancer patients, traumatic brain injury patients, and survivors of natural disasters. A. Nuray Karanci, a psychology professor at the Middle East Technical University in Ankara, Turkey, studied growth in the survivors of the devastating 1999 Marmara earthquake, which killed more than seventeen thousand people. She began asking survivors what negative changes and what positive changes resulted from the earthquake. People told her over and over that the earthquake led them to change their priorities in life. They gave their families more importance than before. Money and material things mattered less. They were more individualistic before the earthquake, and now they wanted to help others. "What I heard in the field is what started me doing research on this," she says. Karanci has gone on to study trauma and growth in many different groups. And, she says, one of the key factors most associated with growth in any group is social support. "If extroverts experience a lot of stress, then it is more likely that they will experience growth, because they are more likely to call for social support," she says. Outgoing people are more likely to share their problems, to ask for help and be willing to receive it, she says.

But not just any kind of support will do. The most effective support comes from those who are willing to allow the trauma survivor to dictate their needs. The friend or family member shouldn't push to talk about things the person is not ready for, nor should they avoid potentially painful topics. "It is a really nuanced thing that depends on the needs of the individual person," says Maguen. Support should help to build up the person's sense of autonomy, says the University of Nottingham's Stephen Joseph. The kind of support that emphasizes dependence, that tells the survivor what to do instead of enabling them to choose their own path, can be counterproductive. Instead, friends and family members need to allow the survivor to find their own path, to support them in that effort and help them rebuild their lives in their own way. Davies was lucky enough to receive an abundance of this kind of open-ended support while she was in the hospital. Her parents were there just for her, expecting and asking for nothing in return, showing unconditional love in a way that completely upended her understanding of her relationship with them.

Yet Davies still faces some struggles in life, and she likely always will. She is torn by her complicated feelings about her late coworker

Claassens. Though she feels horrible that he died, she just didn't know him that well and that makes it hard to grieve over him. Sometimes she feels terrible that so much good has resulted from the accident that cost Claassens his life. "At the core of every day, I felt like I owed it to Gustav to do something fantastic and meaningful with my life," she says. A few minutes later, though, she adds, "My journey was really about my parents."

She faces daily physical challenges, too. Davies is able to walk, but she will never run again, something she misses. Because of the accident she must wear a colostomy bag, which is a constant reminder of her accident. "I still get down about things. I still get upset that I have to wear crap knickers that aren't sexy because they have to hold my bag in. This is horrible, I hate it," she says. "But it's not the end of the world." She was recently diagnosed with arthritis in her left leg and ankle, which were broken in the accident. "I could almost feel myself getting depressed about it, and I thought, It's not that restricting right now. There are things I can do. There are positives, like the fact that I haven't been in a lot of pain in a long time," she says.

Today she and John live in a small house with a garden on a quiet dead-end street not far from the tube stop where she was hit—a place she avoided for many years. Davies is thoughtful and remarkably open. She smiles and laughs easily. To watch her walk, one would never know that she has been through any kind of accident, let alone getting hit by a speeding tube train. The only telltale sign is a tiny scar in the middle of her neck left from the tracheotomy.

Davies and John were married in 2012. Their living room is plastered with wedding photos. "Marriage Rocks" is written on a heart-shaped blackboard hanging in the room. John, a tall, lanky musician with blond dreadlocks, says that Davies is a very different person than she was before the accident. Though they dated for years, he says he never could have married her then. She was all over the place, he thought, and didn't know what she wanted. "I've always loved her, but before the accident she was chaos," says John. "Today she is constantly striving to better herself. When you are with someone who is bettering themselves, for themselves or for others, you are with someone who is constantly going to be changing for the good."

Sitting in the garden behind her home on a bright spring morning with just a few wisps of clouds high above in the blue sky, Davies reflects on all the good that has come from the accident. "I love the outlook I have on life. I value the relationships with people that are in my life," she says. "The accident has made me the best version of me."

Gratitude Inspires Change

Samantha Watson was also in her twenties when her life was upended. Watson was in the middle of her senior year at Brandeis University, just outside Boston. Though she was interested in helping others, perhaps through working at a nonprofit organization—she had volunteered at a domestic violence shelter—she didn't have any more direction than the average college senior. Over the previous five years she had flare-ups of pain in her knee about once a year. But doctors could never find the cause. They kept telling her that it must be bursitis and would give her a cortisone shot and send her on her way. Finally she pressed the issue and received a bone scan. At the time she was focused on classes and grades and the massive impending changes that would lie ahead when she graduated. She didn't think much about the scan. Then, just after Christmas in 1999, she got the results: she had Ewing's sarcoma.

Cancer was not an unheard-of topic in her home. Her mother

was a nurse at Memorial Sloan Kettering Cancer Center in New York City who worked with lymphoma patients, and Watson had been visiting her mother there since she was little. Now Watson needed surgery to remove the tumor that had embedded itself in her tibia. Doctors planned to remove a section of the bone and replace it with a piece of cadaver bone, which would be held in place by screws and metal plates. She would have four rounds of chemotherapy followed by surgery and then another three rounds of chemotherapy. For reasons that Watson can't really explain, she was relatively unfazed by the diagnosis. She understood little about what she was going to face or the risks. "I didn't doubt that I would survive because I really had no clue that I could die," she says. She had a remarkable support group of friends and family. She remained blissfully unaware that her life was riding on the flip of a coin—for a patient of Watson's age, Ewing's sarcoma has a survival rate a little better than 50 percent.

"I was incredibly lucky. I had a zillion people around me from treatment and diagnosis to the biopsy. Whether I was in the house or not, throwing up, taking medications, feeling horrible, there were a lot of people around," says Watson. "I tried to not take it for granted."

But Cynthia Eisenstein, Watson's mother, was very concerned. "When she was growing up, if she got a mosquito bite, life was terrible. If she fell off her bike, she'd cry for three days. These thoughts were in my mind when she was newly diagnosed," says Eisenstein. "I kept thinking, How is she going to do this?"

Watson did survive, and though the recovery was slow and chemotherapy was taxing—she lost her hair and dwindled to around one hundred pounds—she persevered. "When I went through treatment, I had blinders on. I just did what I had to do. I think the cancer treatment was harder on my parents than it was on me. I just had to go through it," she says. "They had to watch me go through it."

Watson tried going to support groups but found them unhelpful. "I was the youngest by a decade and just didn't fit into the groups," says Watson. "I was in a totally different life stage. I wanted to talk about going back to college and dating and starting a career."

Watson went back to school a year later to finish her last semester. It was a rough transition. She was living in a suite with six juniors—normal twenty-year-olds, concerned about papers and tests and the minutiae of college life. Watson knew they were good people, but she had a hard time relating. "I thought, Wait a second, my perspective has changed. I had a better sense of what was important to me," she says. At the same time, she found herself struggling to keep up with her school schedule. She was tired all the time. She didn't have the energy to focus. She missed classes because she was too exhausted to get out of bed. She was sick a lot. Something was clearly still wrong.

Her doctor ran blood tests. The results were bad. The chemotherapy had caused her body to begin making new cancer cells. This was a different kind of cancer: myelodysplastic syndrome, or MDS, a precursor to leukemia that occurs in a tiny percentage of Ewing's sarcoma survivors. The disease was serious and had progressed significantly and Watson would need a bone marrow transplant if she was going to survive. She was worried, far more fearful than she was with her previous bout of cancer. A five-year-old boy that she had been friends with on the cancer ward had died after his bone marrow transplant. She knew that this time she might not make it.

In order to get the bone marrow transplant, Watson needed to have aggressive chemotherapy, far more powerful than anything she had experienced with her Ewing's sarcoma. Doctors needed to first move the cancer back to stage 1 and then cripple her immune system so that her body wouldn't be able to reject the new bone marrow. She had been staying with her mother in Vermont in August 2001 when she got the call that she needed to come to New York to begin the treatments. Her mother packed the car and waited for Watson. But she wasn't coming downstairs. Her mother went up to check on her. "She was just sitting there," says Eisenstein. "I asked her what was going on. She said, 'I don't know if I'll ever see my room again.'"

The treatments were terrible. She threw up a lot. She lost her hair, again. She developed painful sores in her mouth and high fevers. "It was frightening," says her cousin Leslie Stern, who watched Watson fight for her life. "It brought her to the brink of death."

Stern came down to New York from Boston often. "There were always like twenty people in the waiting room," says Stern. "People came out of the woodwork; there was a strong web of people rooting for her. It was incredible and it went on for a long time." Watson's father and her mother were both there for her every day. Sometimes friends would talk; other times they would just sit quietly. A friend who was in medical school would just sit in Watson's room and study. Watson says the support was central to her ability to handle what she was going through. "I was never alone in the room," says Watson. "It also, in a strange way, normalized what I was going through. It was so public. If I had to take a shower or use the bathroom or throw up or any number of gross things, it was a big group effort."

Despite complications with the bone marrow donation—the sample was very small—her transplant took. But recovery was a long and slow process. She needed two or three transfusions a day and her friends and family stepped up, dropping off food, helping with expenses, and most important, donating blood and platelets. A friend's father went as often as he was allowed, even though the woman who took the platelets was not known for her painless touch. "A few times that lady really butchered him, and he kept coming," says Watson. "There is something so personal about blood, you probably can't get more personal—it went out of their body and into mine."

In November, more than two months after she went into the hospital, Watson was told that her immune system was strong enough and that she could leave. "I broke down," she says. "I was too afraid to leave the hospital."

She spent the next year in a Manhattan apartment with her mother, recuperating and waiting for her immune system to get robust enough for her to go outside and reengage with the world. Her days mostly consisted of sleeping, taking pills—forty-six a day—throwing up, and trying to eat. At the age of twenty-three she was under a kind of house arrest with her mother. "I watched my friends graduate, get their first jobs, go on dates, get their own apartments; they were all moving on and I was stuck inside and not doing anything," says Watson.

Watson moved back to Boston in September 2002 to start school again. Seven months later she went to a conference for young adult survivors of cancer. "It was like I was hit over the head," says Watson. "It was a moment of clarity." She discovered an entire group of people who were struggling with the same issues that she faced. Right away she knew that she was going to devote herself to helping them. "For me that was the biggest transition point—from being overwhelmed and sad and scared, all these bad things, to a place where I could channel all of that into something positive."

Watson launched Surviving and Moving Forward: The SAM-Fund for Young Adult Survivors of Cancer in 2003. But she quickly realized that she lacked the knowledge to run the organization the way she wanted. In 2005 she went to graduate school for a master's degree in nonprofit management to learn how to successfully run the SAMFund. The organization raises money to help young people recover financially from cancer and distributes small grants to young adults with cancer to help with bills and student loan payments. In the organization's first decade it distributed more than $1.1 million in grants to young adult cancer survivors and provided thousands of people with information and online support.

Watson was able to conceive of this organization only because she had cancer. And, without the support of friends and family, it's unlikely that she would have launched the SAMFund at all, let alone sustained it for so long. She did so because she felt like she owed it to each of those people who had selflessly helped her to do something meaningful with her life. "At the end of the day I needed to do this, to pay it forward. There is no way to say thank you for that kind of support," says Watson. "There are so many ways that they saved my life, made my life better. There are so many times that you say thank you in a day. If a waiter brings you a glass of water you say thank you. That is not in the same stratosphere. I needed to do something and I think good actions speak louder than words. I don't have any words to show how grateful I am, so this is how I show it, how I pay it forward. It is my responsibility to do it."

All of the social support from friends and family, all of the things these people did, large and small, to help Watson left an incredible impression on her. She was able to move her focus away from her own illness and outward toward everyone who took time away from their own lives to help her. That in itself is a remarkable step. She had plenty to be upset about and no one would fault her for being depressed, angry, bitter, stewing in the horrible unfairness of being struck by cancer twice in her very young life (and in a cruel and ironic twist, the treatment for the first cancer actually caused her second cancer). Though she certainly wasn't happy about this—it was painful and scary and she felt as if the world had moved on and left her behind—there was something about the support that moved her, that pushed her outward and got her thinking about what she might do when she was healthy again. She was driven by gratitude for the help that she received.

Gratitude is an important area of interest in positive psychology. Researchers have found it so tied up with well-being that Martin Seligman, the director of the Positive Psychology Center at the University of Pennsylvania and a leading proponent of positive psychology, has developed elaborate exercises to foster feelings of gratitude. He has individuals write letters to those who have influenced them in life that explain how the relationship has helped them and why they are grateful. Then the people must deliver the notes by hand and wait while the person reads it. That will likely turn into a meaningful discussion about the relationship and gratitude. He found that those who tried this gratitude visit reported large decreases in depression and large increases in happiness. Gratitude is an important step toward well-being.

But what about post-traumatic growth? In Watson's case, her large social network was crucial to her ability to handle her cancer treatments. They helped her reenter the world and understand all the ways in which this experience changed her. Just as Davies's family support helped her, Watson's support network—her parents, her family, and friends—was a vital part of helping her to heal, to avoid the worst post-traumatic stress symptoms, and to help her use the terrible circumstances of her cancer as an opportunity to look for something meaningful to do with her life.

For Watson, the support she received quickly transformed into gratitude for that support. And the overwhelming feeling that she owed those who helped her, that she should in turn help others just as she had been helped, changed her life. Gratitude pushed her to find a new direction for herself, to live her life differently, with others in mind, to reach out and to help.

Chiara Ruini, an Italian psychologist, has been researching just this phenomenon. She is a clinical psychologist and an associate professor at the University of Bologna in Italy. She spent a summer at Seligman's Positive Psychology Center and teaches the only university-level positive psychology course in Italy. She has been researching post-traumatic growth because of the stories that she hears from her clients who have survived cancer. And, given how important gratitude is to positive psychology, she was curious if it played the same role in growth. But rather than simply look at gratitude as an emotion, a temporary feeling set off by something like the gratitude exercise, she was curious about the relationship between people who are predisposed to gratitude—those who readily see the effort that others are making around them and want to pay them back in some way—and growth. "I wanted to measure gratitude as a predisposition, a general attitude of being thankful for people around you, the good things you receive in life," says Ruini. "My idea was that this predisposition would be associated with more positive adaptations or attitudes, especially during a cancer diagnosis."

Ruini had seventy breast cancer survivors fill out questionnaires that were designed to measure their predisposition toward gratitude, their well-being, mental and psychical health, as well as post-traumatic growth. Ruini found that gratitude was strongly linked to better health and psychological well-being. "People who are more grateful will develop less depression or anxiety when they go through an illness," says Ruini. And gratitude was very strongly correlated with post-traumatic growth, particularly when it comes to changes in spirituality and appreciation for life. "If you are grateful, you realize how many positive things there are in your life and maybe through this acknowledgment and awareness, you have better post-traumatic growth," says Ruini.

As Ruini found, gratitude can be helpful to fostering post-traumatic growth. But gratitude can also be its own kind of growth, a way of appreciating life, of finding a new way to be closer to friends and family. "People become more grateful, and that's a change in priorities, a change in perspective in life," says Stephen Joseph. So on the one hand gratitude can help to facilitate growth. And on the other hand it is a kind of growth in itself.

Watson's changes have been intimately tied up in how the support she received from those around her made her feel. And her changes have been dramatic. Her mother has been completely amazed at the transformation. "I remember thinking, Regardless of the outcome, nothing will ever be the same," says Eisenstein. "I can tell you, it is not the same. It is extraordinary." She was surprised that her daughter started the SAMFund and is amazed at her focus and tenacity. Her father, Glenn Eisenstein, says that his daughter never had a strong sense of what she wanted to do in life. But after her trip to the young adult cancer survivors group in 2003, everything changed. "That was the first time I heard her say, 'I know what I want to do,'" he says.

For Watson, like so many, her growth has not been about happiness. She still struggles with survivor's guilt. Many friends she made in the cancer ward died, including a woman who was about her age. "We are still close to her family and every time I see them I want to cry," she says. "They came to my wedding and I was so happy to have them there and so guilty that I got to do this and their daughter didn't." She gets angry when, aware of how much good she has done with her foundation, someone tells her, "Everything happens for a reason." What is the reason that her friends died? she thinks.

For her, growth has really been about finding meaning in something terrible and trying to pay back those who helped her. Getting all of that love and support at just the right time helped her to move forward in life. She wants to help others who are suffering with cancer but don't have the same deep well of friends and resources. With help, hopefully they, too, can find a positive way forward for themselves. She also pays back in small ways. She has become friends with her bone marrow donor and cherishes those close to her.

For Watson, simply living a good and full life is one of the best ways to pay everyone back. She is now married with two children. Her mother, Cynthia Eisenstein, says that they both know how lucky they are. "Often we will be in a moment with her children and we'll catch each other's eye and we know. Sam knows, deep down in her heart, what could have been." And knowing how close she came to not making it, how much others helped her, just adds more value to her life today. "It is meaningful to me, and hopefully a big sign to people who helped me that I am okay," she says. "I am grateful to have a happy life. I am well and I am married to a wonderful guy and have two awesome kids and I try to make the most of the time I have and to take care of myself and other people."

CHAPTER 6

Expressing Yourself

Growth Requires Honest Communication

In August 2006, Karina Hollekim sat squeezed in among friends in a tiny Cessna as it climbed high above the shore of Lake Geneva in Switzerland. The Norwegian professional extreme skier and BASE jumper and a half dozen similarly employed friends had been invited to perform a group jump in wingsuits, which would allow them to arc through the sky like birds, high above a crowd gathered for the Paragliding World Cup in Villeneuve, Switzerland.

This exhibition was a well-needed break from the high-risk jumps off cliff faces they often performed for film shoots. Here, with no nearby rock faces, trees, or jagged outcroppings to avoid, there were no nerves—it was the kind of jump they each had done hundreds of times before. As the plane ascended, circling high above the meadows and alpine peaks, Hollekim realized that she was living the life she'd wanted ever since she was a teenager—traveling the world, competing in sports she loved. As she looked at her friends, laughing, anticipating the rush of the jump, the freedom of flight, she thought, I am the luckiest woman in the world.

Once they reached the right spot, Hollekim's friends each leapt from the plane. And then it was her turn. She jumped out the door and was soon racing forward at more than ninety miles an hour in her wingsuit.

Then, one by one her friends opened their parachutes. Hollekim opened hers, too. But when she pulled the brake toggle to slow her descent, the lines tangled. The right half of the chute crumpled and she began to spin. Like a human helicopter blade, Hollekim was whipped around in a circle almost parallel to the ground. She had lost friends in accidents just like this. She knew she needed to act fast if she was going to save her life.

She was too close to the ground to cut the chute and deploy the backup, so she tried banking toward the water. But it was no use. Though the partially open chute slowed her fall, nothing she did changed her trajectory or stopped the spinning. The ground approached. She hurtled directly at a boulder.

When Hollekim was four years old, she, her father, and her mother were in a car accident. Her mother was paralyzed in the crash and suffered brain damage. Hollekim was raised by her father, Bjørn Sønsterud, who gave her an early introduction to adventure sports. He was a rock climber and skier who often took his young daughter climbing with him. He was also a strict parent, which didn't mix well with his daughter's rebellious impulses. When she was fourteen years old she moved out to live with a relative. She began competing in extreme skiing events and by twenty-one she was crowned the Nordic free-ride champion. Soon she was traveling the globe to compete and appear in films.

In 2000 she met Jeb Corliss, an American BASE jumper, and

traveled to Idaho to learn how to hurl herself off cliffs and bridges and how to fly in a wingsuit. She had found her sport. "I loved it. I craved it. It became addictive," she says. She quickly cultivated a reputation as a highly motivated perfectionist willing to take risks in front of the camera and was traveling three hundred days a year to film and compete. Each time she would master a jump or ski a particularly harrowing mountain face, she would push herself to go further. She jumped off the Jin Mao Tower in China, a 1,380-foot-tall office building. She and a friend climbed to the top of Kaga Tondo, a 3,800-foot-tall spire in the remote Mali desert and did the first wingsuit jump off its top. Her turbulent relationship with her father contributed to her obsession. "I had to fill that empty space with something," she says. "So I filled it with BASE jumping, something that made me happy."

As her adventure sports career took off, her father—with whom she'd reconciled years earlier—and her lifelong friend Anne Romsaas worried about the escalating danger of her exploits. Ever-riskier jumps were becoming her only priority in life. Even fellow BASE jumpers began to worry. "I had the feeling that she had a point to prove, that she deserved all of this," says Corliss. "When I saw her going down that path, I knew she was not going to stop until she died."

Corliss was almost right. The sport nearly killed her. When Hollekim hit the boulder that day in Switzerland, everything went black. She opened her eyes and saw her legs, twisted and bent 180 degrees from where they should be. She thought she must be dead. Then came the pain, an overwhelming, deep pain unlike anything she had felt before—a horrible confirmation that she was alive.

Two days later she woke in the hospital alone and disoriented. Her doctor explained that she had shattered both legs. The right leg suffered twenty-one compound fractures—breaks where the bone comes through the skin. The left had been fractured in four. "You'll never walk again," he told her.

"That just knocked me down. It was unreal, incomprehensible—to not be able to walk. I used my body for everything, for skiing and BASE jumping. All of that was taken from me," Hollekim says. "I just lay there for hours by myself crying."

Hollekim's father flew to Switzerland right away. In the hospital, he stayed up at night pushing the button that would feed his daughter more morphine so she wouldn't wake from the pain. During the day he did his best to hide his own fears, devising ways to keep her spirits up and his mind off the challenges to come. They had parties with her friends who came to visit; they talked about even the tiniest positive development that day. Hollekim was terrified that she would be confined to a wheelchair—a fate that scared her more than death. Sønsterud had watched Karina's mother struggle with paralysis. His own father had been paralyzed by polio. "Karina was not going to handle it well, being in a wheelchair," he says.

Surgeons put a rod in her left leg, the one with only four breaks. The right side became a hodgepodge of plates, screws, and bone grafts so complex that Hollekim doesn't even know how much metal is in that leg. They kept long incisions open for days at a time as they went in and out for more surgeries.

Despite the progress, she was plagued by infections. Three months after the accident she woke in the middle of the night to a wet bed. She turned on the lights and found blood everywhere—soaking the mattress, dripping onto the floor. When the nurses opened her bandages, Hollekim could see through to the bone. An infection had caused the wound to burst open. "I realized that everything was deteriorating—my physical condition, my leg. I could see on the faces of the doctors and nurses that they had lost control and they were scared," says Hollekim. "I just wanted to get home safe and I suddenly realized that might not happen." Doctors tried one more surgery that night and found the cause of the infections—a tiny wad of grass and gravel deep in her leg. The infection cleared up. A month later she finally left the hospital.

She and her father returned to Oslo, where she was admitted to an inpatient rehabilitation facility. This should have been a turning point for her—finally she was out of the hospital, out of danger of losing her leg, even dying. This was the start of her road to recovery. But here things only grew worse. On the first night the facility's founder gave a speech about living with disability. The talk, the room full of amputees and wheelchair-bound people, was too much for her. "It was a shock," says Hollekim. "I realized that I was one of them. I was that person in the wheelchair. I'd never walk again. This was my life now." She was almost immobile. Just sitting upright for a few minutes took so much effort it made her sick. "I just didn't have the strength to fight," she says.

Hollekim sank into depression. She cried, calling her father and asking why she should bother with rehabilitation. Like many people in this situation, Hollekim was tempted to withdraw, to bury her head in sorrow and bitterness. If there was ever a time to spiral, this was it. It is normal and natural to feel victimized, to ask, "Why me?"

Luckily, she had something working in her favor: her father and her friends, a community of people who rallied around her and supported her. Her father, with whom she had had a fractious relationship for much of her youth, was now a key source of strength. He was with her every step of the way, helping to buoy her spirits and keeping her positive. Her BASE jumping and skiing competitors also kept up their visits and calls. All of these people kept her talking, and by extension they kept her engaged with their lives and her own. They never gave her a chance to withdraw. "They were my everything; they gave me hope and strength to get up in the morning and fight," Hollekim says. "They had such belief in me, I didn't want to disappoint them."

And she saw an outpouring of support from a fan base she wasn't really aware of. "After my accident people contacted me from all over the world, lots of people that I had never met but who told me how I had made a difference in their lives and how they wanted me back in the mountains where I belonged," she says. "The fact that I had such an impact on other people's lives just by following my heart and pursuing my dream came as a shock to me."

The Transformative Power of Communication

As much as close relationships can help ward off the worst post-traumatic stress symptoms, and even help one on the path toward growth, what is equally important for so many people is the kind of communication that comes with such support. Research shows that talking about trauma is an important step in healing from trauma, and that keeping emotions in has negative effects. One study found that victims of violent assault who kept the event secret from others were significantly more likely to have adverse health problems than those who spoke about it. Another even found that keeping a traumatic event secret from a strong social network leads to more dysfunction than not having a social network at all.

But communication can do far more than simply help ward off the worst post-traumatic stress symptoms. Talking, writing, and expressing oneself, researchers have found, is central to enabling the kind of deliberate rumination and narrative reframing that is required for growth.

Hollekim was in incredible physical pain, to be sure, but she also faced a remarkable amount of fear and uncertainty about her future. With her legs taken from her, who could she become? At age thirty-one, her entire identity was being challenged. Hollekim's lifelong friend, Romsaas, came to visit her in rehab often and they talked for hours about the kinds of things that longtime friends always talk about—relationships, Romsaas's kids, and endless inconsequential things that make for diverting conversation. Hollekim enjoyed helping her friend navigate even the little frustrations of daily life; it made her feel useful. And, from time to time, they discussed the one thing that scared Hollekim the most: her future. Skiing, flying in a wingsuit, everything she had known was taken from her. She had to reimagine herself and that scared her. She talked about it with Romsaas and her father.

Hollekim was also granted plenty of time to just think, in the hospital, in rehab, through the years of surgeries and rehabilitation, in endless hours in waiting rooms. "I thought about who I was and what kind of value I have to other people. I used to think that other people valued me for my achievement, but that wasn't right. They valued me for who I was," she says.

Thanks to her father's efforts to orient her toward even the smallest positive development, Hollekim realized that, despite all that she'd been through, she could still be happy. She found joy in her friends, in a quiet moment watching the snow fall, when she listened to Romsaas when she needed to talk. She began making lists of these things, tallying up the small moments when she just felt good, which helped her to keep focused on her painful recovery. She also wrote emails to friends, competitors, and her sponsors over the course of many years giving updates on her progress. In one, written in October of 2006 while she was in the rehabilitation facility, she wrote, "An accident like this does something to you. It moves you, it frightens you and it makes you pensive. And in the end I hope it makes you stronger! . . . I've now spent two and a half months in the hospital and it has been the toughest time of my life so far. After 15 surgeries I've never felt more weak or helpless. Recovering from a situation like this makes you wonder about what's important in life. It makes you realize how dependent you are on your friends when it really matters." Even in these emails she tried to find some positive event to relate: though she couldn't move her leg, she could wiggle her toes, an uptick in her weight, increased mobility in her knee, being able to use both legs on the exercise bike. "Writing those letters also became a kind of therapy and I believe it shaped my attitude towards my own situation and healing. It was important for me to appear positive and to implement a kind of hope in those updates," she says. "I'm not sure if this was important in order to persuade myself or because I wanted to protect my readers from the crucial facts, but it helped me."

Over the course of months and years, Hollekim's perspective began to shift. Communicating with those she was closest to helped her to see that she was more than an athlete, that being the best at her sport wasn't the only thing that gave her life importance. "Before the accident, if you asked me if I would ever wind up in a wheelchair, I would have said, 'Shoot me.' Everything I did, everything I loved was physical and if that was ever taken from me, I would not want to live anymore," she says. But now she saw her life differently. "That actually wasn't the worst-case scenario. Realizing that I was much more than a functional body, that was a very good moment."

Through talking, observing, and writing, Hollekim had begun the process of deliberate rumination that Tedeschi and Calhoun see as central to growth. And that set her on a course that required her to rethink who she was, to take into account how the trauma had changed her, stripped her of her identity as an elite athlete and forced her to begin the search for a new way of understanding herself.

Psychologists have found that just this kind of emotional expression can help lead to growth. One study conducted on breast cancer survivors and their spouses in Philadelphia over a year and a half found a correlation between increased emotional expression and growth. Those who did not express their emotions experienced less growth or did not grow at all. The study's lead author, Sharon Manne, a professor at Robert Wood Johnson Medical School at Rutgers University, says that of the 162 couples in the study, those who had the closest relationships were the ones where both spouses reported growth. And in the counseling work that she does with couples where one spouse has cancer, the closeness of the relationship, how much the couple can talk openly and honestly about the experience, and the extent to which they think of the cancer as something that they are both experiencing can make it more likely that both spouses will report positive change.

Researchers have also found that women are both more likely to grow than men from a traumatic experience and that when they do grow, they actually report higher levels of positive change than men. Richard Tedeschi and Lawrence Calhoun, who pioneered this field of study, along with their coauthors examined this by reviewing seventy separate studies that broke down growth along gender lines. Across nearly all of these studies women were more likely to report growth than men. And they reported higher levels of growth than male trauma survivors. One of the reasons may be that women are often more at ease expressing emotions and seeking support from friends and family than men are—according to the stereotype, to be sure, but also according to some research. "Women are more likely to express what they are going through inside than men," says Calhoun.

"And I'm willing to bet that they are also more skilled at responding in a helpful way."

Hollekim's physical recovery took years of painful rehabilitation and twenty surgeries. It wasn't until a year after arriving in rehab that Hollekim attempted her first steps in a chest-high walker. With much of her weight supported by the walker, she stood and inched across her room and down the hall on legs so atrophied that her knees bulged wider than her thighs. The nurses and doctors stopped and stared in disbelief. One nurse hugged her and started crying. Finally, sixteen months after the accident, she had started to walk.

The Power of Writing

About six months later, Hollekim was asked to give a speech about her recovery to 1,500 people. She accepted immediately. Then she realized what she had done. She had never spoken in public before and she was terrified. But with support from her friend Romsaas, Hollekim set about writing her speech. The exercise forced her to reflect on who she had been, what she had been through, and where she might be headed. It forced her to think about her life's narrative, both her old narrative before the accident and what her new narrative might be. "Writing it all down, telling the story the way I wanted to tell it, it became almost therapy," she says. "By writing it all down I was able to sort out my thoughts."

Standing before a roomful of strangers and revealing her intimate fears and struggles, her uncertain hopes for the future, was terrifying. "Saying out loud simple words like 'ten seconds later my life changed forever' almost made me start crying," says Hollekim. "I had never said those words out loud before and I realized then that my life had changed forever." When the crowd stood and applauded, Hollekim felt goose bumps. When people came up to her after her speech and told her how much they connected with her story, she discovered something new: her accident and ongoing recovery had taken on a depth of meaning that it never had before. She realized that her story, her struggle, was something anyone could identify with. What she had suffered through could help others who were also suffering. She understood that she was much more than an athlete. She got a glimpse of a new possibility for who she might be and how she might remake her future.

Writing played a crucial role in helping Hollekim to remake herself. And a large body of research shows that writing can be remarkably helpful for people recovering from trauma. In fact just the slightest bit of writing promotes a broad range of benefits. It's an entire therapeutic approach and field of inquiry that was started almost by accident.

Several decades ago, James Pennebaker, who is now the chair of the psychology department at the University of Texas at Austin, was having problems with his marriage. One day he sat down and wrote about what he was feeling. He never gave what he wrote to his wife. He didn't even keep it. He just threw the paper out. But shortly afterward he noticed something strange. He felt better.

Pennebaker didn't think too much about it but over the next few years, whenever something upsetting happened, he would just sit down and write about it. Then he began looking at the research around trauma and communication. While it was clear that there were real benefits to be gained from communicating with others in the wake of traumatic experience, he felt that engaging others also left a lot to chance. Much of the value of the communication was in how the expression was received by the person the trauma survivor was talking to. Was the survivor dismissed? Did the listener change

the subject or make an unpleasant face? Was the listener open and accepting? If things did not go well, the value of the conversation could
be diminished. "What if you could take away all of that uncertainty
in the face-to-face communication and the person just wrote down
their thoughts?" he wondered.

Pennebaker devised an experiment in which students would
write about a traumatic experience for fifteen minutes, four days
in a row. One group would do so just recounting the facts of the
event, without any emotion or personal reflection. The other would
write about the emotions and meaning of the event. He asked those
writing about the meaning of the event to dig deep into their emotions and to think about how the trauma affected their relationships
with friends and family, how it changed who they are and what they
wanted from life. They had to write continuously for the fifteen-
minute period. He assured them that whatever they wrote would be
confidential.

The results surpassed any of Pennebaker's expectations. Those who
wrote only about the facts reported no changes in any area of their
lives. Those who wrote about the meaning of the traumatic event and
the emotions triggered reported significant changes. They had fewer
visits to their doctors in the following months and used less aspirin
than the other group. They also reported back that the experiment
was beneficial over time. "Months after the first experiment students
would come up to me on campus and say, 'Thank you for letting
me be in your study,'" he says. "Clearly it was bringing about some
meaningful things."

That was the beginning of a long line of studies that Pennebaker
conducted using this technique, which he calls expressive writing (he
has also written books on the subject). Pennebaker began looking at
both the psychological benefits and the physical health benefits as

well. For one study published in 1995, he collected blood samples from forty medical students. He randomly assigned them to either write about their traumatic experiences or to write about unrelated control topics over the course of four days. Then they were given hepatitis B vaccines and later boosters. Blood was collected before each booster and at six months after the initial shot. He found that those who had written about their traumatic experience had significantly higher levels of antibodies in their blood than those who wrote about unrelated topics.

Since his first 1986 study, other researchers have conducted hundreds of studies on expressive writing. One review of studies on expressive writing published more than ten years after Pennebaker's original paper found that these simple writing exercises had significant psychological and physiological benefits, and subsequent meta-analyses have generally agreed. Studies have found that expressive writing reduced blood pressure during writing and that blood pressure stayed down for months afterward; that students who used expressive writing showed an improvement in their grades. It even helped job seekers get hired more quickly than those who did unrelated and superficial writing. Even expressive writing for two minutes two days in a row has been shown to have some benefit. One of the keys, Pennebaker says, is that this particular kind of writing is only for the subjects, not to be shared with anyone. "You are not putting on a show for anyone else," says Pennebaker. "You have to be honest with yourself; otherwise why the hell are you doing it?"

Why does this seemingly simple process work? Pennebaker says that these traumatic experiences tend to remain in the victim's awareness until they are either made sense of cognitively, or they simply fade with time. Making sense of trauma—understanding it and coming to terms with what it means—is a relatively efficient way of comprehending and accepting adverse experience. Waiting for a trauma to fade away can take an awfully long time and lead to lots of problems. By talking or writing about difficult experiences, survivors are forced to translate them into language, which is particularly important with traumatic memories. Life-threatening events activate the amygdala, the brain's fear center. Those memories are red hot with emotion but can lack language and context. Writing helps survivors to label the experience, attaching language to it that allows survivors to understand and process the event instead of leaving it as some alert adrift in our neural wiring. Once that's done, people can assign it meaning, some level of coherence, and give the event a structure and place in their lives. Representing the experience with language is a necessary step toward understanding the experience, Pennebaker argues.

Writing, Pennebaker says, is different than talking to someone. It forces a person to really think through an event and its consequences in a more detailed and thorough way than just talking about them. That was clearly the case for Hollekim. One study of Pennebaker's randomly assigned students to either express traumatic experience using bodily movement or to express it using bodily movement and writing for ten minutes a day for three days. Only the students who did both the movement and the writing experienced significant improvements in health and grades. The health gains required translating the experience into language, not simply expression of the emotions.

Studies have shown that writing about powerful experiences in an organized way is more beneficial than doing it in a disorganized way, and research shows that while talking is helpful, and one can be forced to organize the experience in a deep and meaningful way in a discussion, writing demands such organization and pushes one to dig a little deeper. "You start asking yourself how this affected me, how it changed my relationship with this person, the way you think about life and death, to see how the major upheaval touched every part of your life," Pennebaker says.

The idea of using writing to help trauma survivors intrigued Joshua Smyth, a psychology professor at Pennsylvania State University. Often trauma survivors are overwhelmed by the memories of their experience. The memories remain deeply emotional and the event itself can seem too large, too powerful to engage with. But writing, he has found, offers a possible solution. "Writing forces you to break ideas and events into smaller units that you can write about," he says. The whole traumatic event may be overwhelming, he says, but in writing one must choose a place to start. Forcing people to write slows them down and provides an opportunity to clearly assess the event piece by small piece.

In a study Smyth conducted that was published in 2008, a group of people who had been diagnosed with severe PTSD (Vietnam veterans and survivors of sexual assault) were divided into two groups. One wrote about time management and the other wrote about their emotional reaction to their traumatic experience—expressive writing. Three months later those who did the expressive writing showed modest improvements in the severity of their PTSD and small decreases in stress indicators like the release of cortisol. And the vast majority of those in the expressive writing group showed a significant amount of post-traumatic growth. The first group did not show any growth at all. Smyth says that writing can help to spur growth, in part because it forces people to construct a story about the trauma and to start to see how the narrative of their lives might change. The University of Nottingham's Stephen Joseph says that asking people to write forces them to create a narrative without being judged. "It helps them construct a story of what happened. They are able to create a sense of coherence and meaning and look into the future," he says. And that process can help to jump-start the kind of deliberate rumination that can lead to narrative reframing, putting one on the path to growth.

And that is exactly the role that writing played for Hollekim. She made notes about the things that made her happy, But she also was forced, by having to write a speech, to examine her own life story. An inspirational speech requires a narrative, and one that features positive change. Hollekim had to dig deep into who she was before the accident; she was forced to think about what the accident had taken from her and how she planned to remake her life afterward. Through writing, Hollekim was forced to focus more on her experience and express all that she had been through in a thoughtful and coherent way that is hard to do when just thinking or even talking—she was exploring her own narrative and ultimately creating a new narrative for herself.

For Hollekim her speech also provided her with a different benefit, one she did not expect. She was able to connect with another community and source of support that would change her life dramatically. "I realized that my life was not about life-threatening experiences anymore," says Hollekim. "It was more meaningful and rewarding and not as selfish." Today she makes her living as a speaker traveling to tell her story and inspire others, something that her father says has helped to make her a new person. "She has turned all of this into something positive," he says. "She has a story to tell and it's important for others to see that it is possible to get up from very low down and to be able to make a life for themselves."

Thankful for the Accident

Three years after her accident Hollekim was walking, but still in constant pain. She had been on painkillers for so long that she had to go through detox twice. Finally she visited the Red Bull Diagnostic and Training Center in Austria, which helps athletes bridge the gap between rehabilitation and training. She received deep tissue massage and relearned the mechanics of walking. She did more weight training. Under her trainer's watch, her muscles began to heal and function properly. And over time the pain began to dissipate. She was getting closer to the goal she set for herself when she began rehab—to get back on skis. The risks were high. Her legs are held together by so many plates and screws that in an X-ray they look like the bargain bin at a hardware store. A simple fall could put her back in the hospital.

In January 2010, three and a half years after her accident, Hollekim went to Hemsedal, a ski area near her father's house. The mountain opened an hour early so she could ski alone. She had been anticipating and dreading this moment for years: hopeful that she could reclaim a part of her identity, terrified that her legs would fail her. In the early-morning darkness, under glaring lights, she eased off the chairlift and slid down the ramp. That first brief glide felt instantly natural—more than walking ever did. Accompanied by her father, her boyfriend, and her physical therapist and with her mother and a group of friends waiting at the bottom, she skied down a groomed intermediate slope. "In that moment, I felt like I was back to being me," she says.

Now Hollekim walks with a near-normal gait. She wears short skirts if she wants, no longer afraid to show legs that are so marked by scars that a stranger once asked if she'd been mauled by a shark. She travels widely still, but now to tell her story to others. And she skis, not just on groomed slopes but slicing through untracked powder in rugged terrain, once again feeling the freedom of the mountains, the snow beneath her feet, the friends by her side. But skiing is a pastime, no longer a career. She has a new career: telling her story of recovery and transformation. "I have grown a lot. I am wiser in my decisions and I appreciate what I have," Hollekim says. "I am thankful it happened."

That is a remarkable statement—to be thankful for such a painful, debilitating, and life-changing accident, particularly for someone who says she was blissfully happy, successful, and fulfilled in her life before. But Hollekim means it. She says that before the accident, she had been driven, a perfectionist, restless and hungry for success. Her father and her friend Romsaas say that as her career progressed, she didn't understand how the risky sports she pursued affected those around her. She traveled constantly, pursuing the life that she loved. But in part it also became a way to escape her problems and insecurities. "If you can master the task of controlling life and death, like it feels like you do when you BASE jump, your everyday problems feel mundane and small in comparison," she says. "This kind of escape gives you energy and strength. You feel empowered and invincible." But of course she wasn't invincible. And because of that today she is different. She is a more attentive friend. She is much closer to her father. She is more responsible and more focused on her important relationships with those close to her. Her old insecurities pale in comparison to all she has overcome. Her new pursuits feed a side of her that she was completely unaware of before the accident. Her new career is meaningful and gives back to others.

Her wingsuit-flying friend Corliss says the change is clear. "When I hang out with her now, I can see it, even my mom can see it, it's like she glows," he says. "She is the happiest I have ever seen her." Hollekim has seen the changes, too. She's more at peace with herself. The restlessness is gone. She appreciates simply being alive, in a way she never did before. "I don't need to fill the void with anything anymore," she says. "The void is gone and I am a happier person today."

CHAPTER 7

Looking for the Positive

The Transformative Power of Optimism

ON A FOGGY MORNING BEFORE SUNUP IN AUSTIN, TEXAS, MATT Cotcher got out of bed and made himself two slices of toast with peanut butter and banana. He ate one and then drove to downtown Austin. With about forty-five minutes to spare—he left early to avoid any traffic that might stress him out—he sat in his parked car relaxing and slowly eating the other slice of toast. Then, as the sun rose through the murky haze that hung around the Texas Capitol, he joined the twenty thousand runners assembling in a sprawling line preparing to run the Austin Marathon.

Cotcher is tall and thin. His head is shaved to a stubble of dark hair, which helps to highlight a pale white scar, about four inches long, that arcs down the back of his head to the base of his neck. As the race began, runners started to lurch forward, and Cotcher disappeared into the mass of slowly bouncing bodies.

He was no favorite to win the race. Nor was there a large group of friends to cheer him on. This was his third marathon in the past year—his second here in his hometown of Austin—and even his friends weren't willing to drag themselves out of bed to see Cotcher off this early in the morning. Nonetheless, it was remarkable that he started this race at all.

In 1991 Cotcher moved to Austin from Atlanta to go to college at the University of Texas. But a few years later he left school without finishing. After a successful decade working for a start-up company in Atlanta, he began thinking about his degree. "I had never failed at much in life, and it was very important for me to go back to UT and correct the biggest failure in my past," he says. After a decade in sales, he was interested in finding a new career. He moved back to Austin in 2005 and reenrolled. "I had a kind of optimism that I could re-create myself professionally," says Cotcher.

Cotcher had always been athletic—he played football and basket-ball growing up in Atlanta—and was a rabid sports fan. He idolized Keith Jackson, a broadcaster who spent forty years with ABC Sports. Now he wanted to become a sportscaster. Texas, with a culture of sports mania spanning from high school football to its championship professional basketball teams, was fertile ground. He quickly landed an internship and later a job with a company setting up deals to stream broadcasts of high school football games online. By the time he graduated from the University of Texas in December 2006, he was doing live commentary for the games and receiving high praise from veteran sportscasters. "I was on the right path to becoming the next Keith Jackson," Cotcher says.

But in the months after graduation, Cotcher was plagued by powerful headaches. Finally, in April 2007, he went to a clinic. As the visit was wrapping up Cotcher stood, stumbled, and nearly fell to the ground—his balance just gave way. The doctor was worried enough to send him out for a CT scan at a nearby hospital. After the scan, doctors followed up with an MRI. The news was not good. A racquetball-size mass was entwined around his brain stem—the part of the brain that controls basic functions like breathing, digestion, heart rate, and communication between the brain and body. This was a particularly terrible spot for a tumor, especially for one so large.

Things moved at an incredible pace. One day he was a happy, normal thirty-five-year-old working on creating a new career for himself. The next he was diagnosed with brain cancer. After consulting with those closest to him, Cotcher opted for the most invasive surgery to ensure that the entire tumor was cut out. This radical surgery decreased the tumor's chances of recurrence, but it also posed real risks—risks that Cotcher didn't entirely understand. "In my mind, having brain surgery was going to be like breaking a bone. I might be out of commission for six to twelve months," says Cotcher. "I was totally normal and functioning perfectly, so why would I think that removing the tumor would do anything other than make my headaches go away?"

Ten days after that first scan, Cotcher was in the hospital getting prepped for surgery. The night before his surgery, he told his best friend, Kevin Shuvalov, that he thought it might take two or three months before he was back to normal. "No one came to him and said, 'Hey, your life is going to change drastically,'" Shuvalov says.

Cotcher was concerned about how the surgery might impact his newfound broadcasting career and talked to the surgeon as he was wheeled into the operating room. "The last thing that I said to the surgeon was, 'Don't wreck my voice,'" says Cotcher.

Cotcher's family and friends and Shuvalov's family, about fifteen people in all, assembled in the waiting room. When doctors began operating they discovered that the tumor was not a solid mass that could be cut into pieces and removed with relative ease. Instead it was more like Jell-O. Each piece they tried to remove broke apart into tiny pieces. The tumor had to essentially be scraped out bit by bit. This made his already invasive surgery far more damaging. "It was beyond rough," says Shuvalov. "The doctors weren't sure he would make it through the night."

Cotcher regained consciousness the next day. And shortly afterward his doctors discovered the first result of the surgery: when they removed Cotcher's breathing tube, he couldn't take a breath on his own. He spent the next few weeks on a respirator with a breathing tube down his throat. Soon other effects of the surgery became clear. "The first time I really remember being frightened was when a speech/swallow therapist came into my room with a cup of crushed ice," says Cotcher. "She spoon-fed me a small piece and asked me to swallow it. I couldn't. I didn't understand why. I just knew that when I was supposed to be swallowing, nothing was happening."

Cotcher's left side was partially paralyzed. He couldn't swallow. He couldn't move many of the muscles in his face. His balance and coordination were impaired. He couldn't walk. Because he couldn't swallow, Cotcher had to use a feeding tube—a tube that is inserted directly to his stomach, bypassing his mouth and esophagus. He was fed by pouring pureed food down the tube. Cotcher had been desperate to get the breathing tube out of his throat so he could talk. It was frustrating to communicate by writing on a small whiteboard—he could think so much faster than he could write and he couldn't converse with friends and doctors. But when the tube came out he was in for another surprise. "Finally the tube came out and my brain didn't know how to talk," Cotcher says. "I wanted to say something and nothing came out. It was very scary."

Cotcher maintained a brave face, but beneath it all he was terrified. "He never once said, 'This really sucks,' " says Shuvalov. "But you could see it in his eyes, you could see him thinking, Holy heck, what am I going to do?"

After a month or so in the hospital, Cotcher was moved into a rehabilitation facility. Nurses stimulated the muscles in his face with tiny electric shocks that forced the muscles to contract, which in turn would stimulate his brain, hopefully helping it to remember how to make the movements. Progress was painstakingly slow and because his cognitive powers were never impacted by the surgery, he was deeply aware of how far he had to go. "I knew the word *cat*," he says. "I could read it. I knew what a cat was; my brain even knew how to pronounce *cat*. My brain remembered everything about cat, but it didn't know how to make me say it. It was the same way with walking, jumping, smiling, breathing. My brain remembered all of those things and I felt like I could do them, but when I tried to perform the task, nothing."

Cotcher had to relearn how to walk. At first he just worked on standing and sitting. Once he mastered that, he walked with the aid of a grocery cart. The cart was replaced by a walker, then he used a cane, then a hand on a rail. Eventually he began walking unaided. "I went from walking to a fast shuffle to loosely jogging down the hall. It was miserable. I was so athletic before. I realized that normal is never going to be what normal used to be," says Cotcher.

The lingering paralysis in his face left his speech slow and slurred. People often thought that he was mentally disabled. "He couldn't walk down the street," says Shuvalov. "When we went to a game, everyone thought he was drunk; he would get jostled in the crowd. He was just all over the place and it was hard for him."

Cotcher would certainly be well within his rights to be angry, depressed, and bitter at this freakish turn of events, at his overwhelming new limitations and the excruciatingly slow pace of recovery. But, he says, through it all he never sank into depression. Instead he remained positive, and he focused on getting better and learning everything he could about his condition and potential treatments. "I believe there are positive-minded people and negative-minded people; you are either one or the other," Cotcher says. "I am a positive person and always have been. If anything, my medical journey has accentuated that fact. Being depressed or bitter or angry just never occurred to me. Rather than be bitter about what I lost, I put that energy into educating myself on why and how things function the way they do. Not only is it a better use of my time, it's also helpful in the long term."

Seeking Out the Positive

Cotcher's attitude, his way of looking at his situation and searching for practical solutions, his refusal to be dragged into negativity, and his innate optimism were all key to his ability to recover and begin to find a new life for himself. "He is very forward-looking, and he has a really positive attitude," says Catherine Whiting, Cotcher's therapist. Cotcher gave her permission to speak about him and how the cancer has impacted his life. "He focuses on the here and now, and on the good parts of the here and now," she says.

A remarkable amount of research indicates that having a positive attitude is helpful in recovery from cancer and for other traumatic events. Sharon Manne, the researcher at the Rutgers Cancer Institute of New Jersey, says that optimists have lots of advantages over others in these situations. They have broad and deep support networks. They are more integrated into their communities. They live longer and have more fulfilling lives. "It's an advantage for everything," she says.

The way one frames a traumatic event, positively or negatively, can have a significant impact on how one recovers from it, says Jane

Shakespeare-Finch. That is not to say that people should pretend that a terrible event is actually great. Instead they need to assess the change that it has brought to their lives and begin to understand how to integrate it with who they are and who they want to be going forward. They need to accommodate the experience in the terms that Jean Piaget and Stephen Joseph use. And the more that one can focus on the positives, to find even the tiniest thing that is beneficial, the better off one will be.

Hollekim, in the previous chapter, did this with the talks she had with her father and the writing she did in her journal and emails— where she identified even the tiniest positive event, like just sitting and watching the snow fall through her hospital window or wiggling her toes. She used her journal, those conversations, and emails to help herself stay focused on positive developments instead of dwelling on the overwhelming and uncontrollable disaster that had befallen her.

Shakespeare-Finch saw this kind of positivity at work when she helped the survivors of the terrifying bushfires in Australia in 2009 that killed 173 people. She worked with the survivors over time, helping them to begin to think of things they may have maintained or gained. For some, the fact that they survived the fires at all or that their children survived could be a starting point for seeing something positive. By comparing their terrible plight to the even worse situation of so many, they could begin to see how they were in fact better off than some. And that might give them a tiny strand of something positive to hold on to. Many saw their communities rally around the survivors and those who had lost homes. Some people chose to cultivate deeper relationships with people who were the most supportive and let go of relationships with others who were not. "There was a positive aspect of all of this in the sense of loyalty that came from the people that were in their lives for a long time," she says.

These people were not ignoring the trauma or pasting it over with a veneer of cheer. They understood what they had lost and the struggle they were in for, but they also had the capacity to find something positive, to seek it out and give it weight as well. And it is just that kind of attitude that may be the most beneficial. James Pennebaker, the University of Texas psychology professor who pioneered the study of expressive writing, was curious about the role of positive emotion in health. So he decided to go back through a half dozen of his studies to see whether those who conveyed positive emotions in their expressive writing had any health advantages over others. He analyzed the language the subjects used in their writing, looking for positive words like *happy* and *laugh* and negative words like *sad* and *angry.* The language did make a difference. The more positive language subjects used, the more their health improved—positivity was a benefit. But their health did not improve the most. The group whose doctor visits dropped the most were those who used a moderate number of negative emotion words. Those people were expressing their struggles in addition to some sense of positivity, and that mixture, a realistic acceptance of their struggle and a hope for something better, turned out to be the most beneficial.

For Cotcher, his naturally positive attitude not only helped him to recover; it has helped him to reinvent his entire understanding of what he values and how he wants to live his life. Cotcher's life slowed down dramatically. He could no longer work and everything that he did took longer and occurred at a slower pace. That gave him the time to learn about his disabilities with an eye to fixing them. Rather than simply get frustrated about his inability to swallow, Cotcher found out about a possible fix—an implant that could improve his speech and swallowing. He researched online until he found the top specialist at the Mayo Clinic. He emailed with the doctor and soon made his way to Minnesota for two days of tests and evaluation. The doctors recommended several procedures that could improve Cotcher's quality of life and at the end of 2009 he had the surgeries.

Not long afterward, Cotcher began eating, slowly. When Cotcher went over to his friend Shuvalov's home for dinner he would need to start eating long before anyone sat down and he would still be eating long after everyone else finished. That is frustrating and even awkward, but it was far better than pouring pureed food down a tube into his stomach for the rest of his life.

Though Cotcher's thinking was not impaired by the surgery, everything else about his life was. He walks slowly and it has taken him years to learn the balance and coordination necessary to have a normal stride. To this day he still can catch himself teetering backward in the kitchen when doing dishes or cooking. He speaks very slowly and can be hard to understand. He has lost hearing in one ear and it is impaired in the other, making it hard for him to hear his own speech clearly and to talk with others.

Most people would find that slowness frustrating, a point of constant friction in a world where speed and efficiency are valued above all else. Shuvalov says that spending time with Cotcher can be a bit like spending time with an elderly parent, not a friend in the prime of his life. "I would have broken all of the dishes by now," Shuvalov says. "That is the greatest test of his character. He has never taken it out on anyone. He has just tried to get better."

But Cotcher, characteristically, does not see these things as a deficit. Instead he sees real benefits in being forced to live life at a slower pace. "Slowing down means that I am much more present in my life. I appreciate everything that happens around me and all of the people in my life," Cotcher says. "When you are near death, everything seems to crystalize. For me that meant being more aware of who I am, who I want to be, and how I interact with the world around me."

In fact, Cotcher says, these physical changes, which forced him into a radically different role in the world, have given him a perspective on life that more of us could benefit from. "I wish that more people could be as awake and aware as I am without having to go through the medical drama. People worry over such inconsequential things and, more importantly, that worry makes them overlook the truly important things," he says. "I live life the way that most people wish they did. When people make New Year's resolutions about being happier or more appreciative then forgo those resolutions in ten days, well, I live every day according to those resolutions."

Cotcher's optimism permeates everything he does and has certainly been critical to helping him to change. But researchers still have many questions about how optimism relates to growth. Optimism is usually defined as expecting good things to happen in the future. But do those who've been through trauma really expect the future to be better? That simplistic definition of optimism may not align well with the experiences of trauma survivors, says UNC Charlotte's Richard Tedeschi. "[Trauma survivors] are not necessarily expecting positive things to happen, because they have seen how easily terrible things can happen," he says. "So maybe they are better-informed optimists. They expect that life does include terrible things."

And perhaps that is why psychologists who look at the question of optimism and post-traumatic growth have found mixed results. Psychologist Stephen Joseph conducted a review of thirty-nine separate studies that documented positive change following trauma. These studies found that those who reported post-traumatic growth also scored high on scales for optimism and positive framing of experience, as well as other factors. One study conducted on cancer survivors in China and published in 2004 found that a positive outlook is overwhelmingly correlated with growth. But other studies have found only a small relationship between optimism and growth.

Sharon Manne at Rutgers says that focusing on the positive—not necessarily optimism, or the idea that good things will happen in the future, but simply looking for positive things and events in the present—is incredibly helpful for the cancer patients she counsels and studies. "They look for what would be helpful for them; they focus on the positive and push the negative stuff away," she says. While there are many steps to moving from the depths of a post-trauma experience to growth—deliberately ruminating on the problems, the narrative reframing, the need for some level of help and support from loved ones—that all may be for naught without the ability and inclination to find some positive meaning. If everything is negative, then it is hard for people to see the potential benefits, the small and even large positive things that can come from a traumatic experience, and to turn their thoughts toward the future and what kind of life they want to lead.

Lawrence Calhoun has seen this throughout his work. "People who engage in more deliberate thought processes are going to look at their situation and see if there is any way that they can use it in a positive way," says Calhoun. "People who are going to focus more on what they are getting out of something than what they are losing are more likely to grow. That requires a certain amount of optimism and an ability to focus on the positive."

A Problem-Solving Attitude

On the day of the Austin Marathon, runner after runner rounded the last corner at the steps leading up to the Texas Capitol and turned toward downtown, covering the last few blocks to the finish line. Each person's face was contorted in its own way, but each expressed the same thing—excruciating pain and incredible willpower, as if the right contorted grimace were the only means left to keep their dead legs moving. Some athletes limped along, barely making it; others pushed themselves to a full sprint, a last, desperate lunge to finish the race. And then came Cotcher. He's tall, at six feet one, and his stride is long. As he turned the corner and bore down on the finish, little changed. He ran with a powerful and even stride. As he covered the final yards before the finish, the struggling runners around Cotcher looked like their brain stems had been mangled, while he was a picture of poised running technique.

That's remarkable. Five years earlier, he could barely walk and staggered like a wildly drunk man when he did. But Cotcher was used to being athletic and exercising. And the more he exercised the faster he could recuperate. His doctors encouraged him to shuffle, walk, and eventually run. When he taught himself to jog again he did it at the golf course behind his town house. It wasn't because of the scenery, but because he fell down so often that he needed to practice somewhere with a soft place to land. He didn't view his total lack of balance and coordination as a chasm impeding his ability to run. Instead he saw it as a logistical challenge. If he was going to fall down when he ran, he'd better find a place to do it with a soft landing. The golf course's well-maintained greens were perfect.

Cotcher approached running with the same level of focus, dedication, and patience that he applied to his rehabilitation. He began by entering small local races, going as far as he could before walking. The first time he ran a full race was in 2011. A picture of him crossing the finish line of the 5K hangs on the wall of his apartment outside Austin. In early 2012 he started thinking about running a marathon—an incredible mental feat of optimism and confidence given how hard running was for him.

As he started to train, Cotcher discovered another problem. With each stride, he uncontrollably slammed his left foot to the ground. He began to worry that he'd wreck his knee or his hip and wind up with even more problems. His left side had been partially paralyzed after his surgery and though it had recovered significantly, it was not 100 percent. After talking with doctors and a running coach, he discovered the problem. His brain didn't know where his foot was in relation to the ground. He could fix the problem, but only if he focused his attention on where his feet were and where the ground was on each and every stride. So much of the automatic calculus that everyone's brains do for them effortlessly all day long, Cotcher must do consciously over and over again. As a result it is very hard for him to do more than a few things at the same time. When he runs he is concentrating so hard on movement and breathing, balance, and coordination that he can't swallow. He has to spit his saliva out every half mile or so. If he needs to drink or eat while running, as is common in marathons, he has to come to a complete stop until he is done chewing or swallowing.

After nearly two years of training, he started the Livestrong Austin Marathon in February 2013. Cotcher finished in 4:19:28, a great time for anyone running their first marathon, let alone someone who couldn't even walk just a few years earlier. The next fall he ran the Chicago Marathon and in 2014 he was back running the Austin race again. This time he improved his time, finishing in 4:05:09.

Cotcher's approach to running is reflective of so many facets of his personality, says Chris Brewer, the deputy director of external affairs with the Livestrong Foundation and Cotcher's close friend. "Everything that he looks at every day, he is trying to make it significant to him, trying to be as successful as he can in a marathon, increasing how well others comprehend his speech, trying to inspire other people," says Brewer. "In Matt's case, he has just made a choice. He's decided that he's going to look for as many positive aspects of his life as he can. He could easily go the other way and no one would fault him for that at all. For him, I think it really is just a choice."

Since his surgery, Cotcher has started a foundation to raise money and awareness about brain cancer. It's called Hawktober and it urges people to get a Mohawk haircut every October to draw attention to the disease. Cotcher's career has come to an end, at least for now. He's on disability and is skeptical that anyone would hire him. So he started this organization both to help others and to keep him focused and using the skills that he learned both in business and journalism. Cotcher also spends a significant amount of time learning more about the brain, about his deficits and what may be behind them, searching for new surgeries and other approaches that may help him to regain his speech, hearing, movement, balance, all the things that he has lost. He has already undergone a half dozen surgeries to help improve many of these functions, but he's certain that as technologies become more advanced and research about the brain only improves our understanding of its mysteries, better fixes will become available.

Cotcher takes a very practical approach to his cancer, too. He sees it as a problem to be solved (in much the same way he viewed his struggle to relearn how to run) rather than as a purely destructive force that has left him a helpless victim. And that has forced him to engage with the trauma rather than avoid it. Cotcher has researched his cancer and delved deep into neuroscience to better understand what may be causing his deficits and how they might be cured. He is active on message boards, not for emotional support, but because the people in these communities know more about his particular cancer and the lingering effects of tumor removal than anyone else. Cotcher's running, too, has engaged him with his deficits, requiring him to master so much in order to compete.

Whiting says that Cotcher once told her that he is no longer capable of multitasking the way he once could. She had to point out to him how much multitasking running requires. And that made him focus on trying to improve his multitasking abilities while running. Now he recites the ABC's while running, hoping that the challenge will help make more new connections in his brain, which may help him regain new functionality.

This approach to life's challenges—engaging with the issue at hand, accepting its limitations yet searching for practical solutions to those things that can be changed—is called problem-focused coping, and it is related to two personality traits, extroversion and positive emotion, both of which Cotcher has in abundance. A study of forty-one cancer patients conducted in Italy and published in 2011 found that problem-focused coping was a key element that contributed to post-traumatic growth among these patients.

A. Nuray Karanci, the professor at the Middle East Technical University in Turkey, found that problem-focused coping was an important element in predicting post-traumatic growth among survivors of the 1999 Marmara earthquake. "This form of active coping allows you to take support from others and engage in necessary behavior, whatever is meaningful for you," says Karanci. "These people are doing things to increase their self-esteem, which is very important because trauma lowers our self-esteem. This [problem-focused coping] helps to give them a new sense of purpose and self-esteem and they gain a new meaning or make a transformation."

As far as Cotcher has come, he still has plenty of obstacles to confront every day. He is easily overwhelmed by too much stimulus— supermarkets, with their bright lights, bright colors, and infinite choices leave him exhausted. A few days after the marathon, he wrote in an email: "Turns out my body finally wore out after the last 4 days. . . . I ended up with night sweats and a fever for most of the night last night. It's not uncommon for me in a time of extreme fatigue." Eating, while better, is still slow. After he finished the Austin marathon, he joked that it would take him two days to consume the 3,500 calories that he burned during the race.

Though he worries that he may never have children, he treasures the close relationships that he has with his nieces and nephews and his friends' children. When Shuvalov bought his son, Drew, a rifle for Christmas, it was Cotcher who taught him how to shoot it. "Drew listened to him intently, did exactly what he told him to do. He had a few targets that were all over the place but they stayed out there for an hour and he got Drew shooting straight—the pride that swelled up in Matt," says Shuvalov. "He felt that he could still offer something to others."

And, of course there is always the possibility that his cancer could come back. And that is not an abstract worry. He has an MRI every year and doctors found an anomalous spot on his brain. They are unsure if it is scar tissue or a tumor. "I am living with the great unknown, knowing that it could come back at any time," says Cotcher. But even that worry is overshadowed by his positive attitude, his ability to value the present over the future. "I am confident that I am healthy and there is nothing wrong; otherwise I could not run the marathon that I just did, so for me that has to be enough," he says. "If I worry about what could happen five years from now, I would miss today. And I am not willing to make that sacrifice."

While Cotcher was always a positive person, he credits the cancer and the struggles he faced after surgery for teaching him a new and better way to live his life. "From the cancer I learned to stay focused in the present. People want something to make them happy instead of just being happy. This whole experience has taught me that if you wait for something external to make you happy, you are missing the point. It's a choice. You just have to be happy and to be really happy you have to live today, not yesterday and not tomorrow," says Cotcher. "You have to live in the moment because that is what matters and that is what you can control."

CHAPTER 8

Finding Meaning in Faith

The Religious Path to Growth

LOUIS D. BROWN WAS THE KIND OF FIFTEEN-YEAR-OLD WHO FELT like he had to hide his intellect. Brown loved to read so much that he amassed a large collection of books and comics and spent hours in his room lost in *The Adventures of Huckleberry Finn* and *Charlie and the Chocolate Factory*. He played Nintendo and would blow off homework from time to time like any fifteen-year-old. But Brown, unlike most his age, had already mapped out his future. He planned to go to college and then graduate school for an advanced degree in aerospace engineering. Then he planned to become the nation's first black president (that was long before the election of President Barack Obama). These are grand ambitions for any child, but in his Dorchester neighborhood of Boston, they were the kind of goals that got you beat up more often than they made you friends, and so Brown tried to downplay his ambition and smarts.

The early 1990s were a violent time in Brown's neighborhood. Gangs were a fact of life. Dealers openly sold drugs on the street. And shootings were not uncommon. Because of the violence around him,

Brown led a sheltered life. He rarely rode the train or walked through the neighborhood on his own. When he went out he usually got a ride from his parents.

Brown wanted to do something to change that. "Adults blamed children for the violence in the community, and whenever things changed or went right, the adults took the credit," Brown told his mother, Clementina Chery. Brown got involved with a group called Teens Against Gang Violence, which gave him an outlet for his feelings and a way to do something positive for his community. "He found his platform, a group of young people with the same goals and determination to do something positive and to take the myth away about young black males with hoodies," says Chery.

On a December afternoon in 1993, Brown left his house to go to a Christmas party for his antiviolence group. At the same time a group of young men were gathering a few blocks away. Someone fired a shot at the group. They scattered, running for safety. One or more of them fired back. Brown, who was walking to the train on an adjacent street, was hit in the back of the head by a stray bullet. He never regained consciousness. Doctors removed him from life support and he died later that day.

When doctors told Chery the news, she could barely understand what they were telling her. Her son was dead? "It's like a trance; you are hypnotized and moving. I remember driving. I was really upset. Cars and busses were honking. Life was still going on. I remember thinking, How dare they, don't they know what just happened?" she says. "Shock, denial, anger, and rage came over me. The world should stop. My world stopped. Why is the world still going?"

Her friend Patricia Zamor was on her way to buy a Christmas tree with her family when she heard about Brown's death. She dropped everything and came to the house. Zamor's mother and brother had both been murdered. She knew well about sudden and traumatic loss of loved ones. Once the word got out that Brown was dead, people filled their small street offering support. Her sister and other family members came to the apartment. Reporters waited outside. Zamor helped to handle the press, trying to give her friend and family space to grieve. "We were all in a trance," says Zamor. "It was a very tough time; she was just walking in a daze."

Chery had grown up in a very religious Catholic household in Honduras. She and her sister went to Sunday school and the family attended service every week and prayer meetings twice a week. Religion was always a big part of their lives. But when her son was killed, Chery pushed back against her faith and God. "I had left the church angry at my priest, my faith," she says. Chery found it hard to reconcile the murder of her son with the fact that she was living a life that she was taught was good and virtuous. "I went to Mass. I donated. It was the foundation that I had from the time I was a child; you went to church every Sunday, you prayed, you read the Bible," she says. But none of that saved her son. Chery wanted to just pull the curtains closed and stay in bed all day. "I was angry at the world and God and everyone," Chery says. "I blamed myself."

But Chery had two other children to care for. Somehow she had to keep going. She turned once again to the church for support. She had always been close to her priest, so she returned and began talking with him. Soon it became a daily ritual. He gave her books to read and talked to her about her family. They both recognized that she needed to find a way forward. "He helped me to begin to heal, to do the inner work," Chery says. "I had to find a way to balance, to grieve the murder of my son and at the same time be a mother to my two living children."

Chery read the Bible often, looking for solace and meaning. She returned to one particular passage again and again: John 14:27: "Peace I leave with you, my peace I give unto you: not as the world giveth, give I unto you. Let not your heart be troubled, neither let it be afraid." It was a sentiment she tried to integrate into every part of her life.

God, she decided, had not abandoned her. He was with her. He was giving her the strength to survive, to be able to move forward and to be there for her family.

Faith Is a Touchstone for Transformation

Stories of trauma, struggle, and transformation can be found in almost every world religion. For those facing terrible tragedies like Chery, these stories can help to provide a guide, another narrative to consider as they face their own crisis and loss, says Kenneth Pargament, a psychology professor at Bowling Green State University in Ohio who has spent his career considering the role that faith plays in trauma recovery and growth. "The stories that stick with us are hopeful stories, not ones of despair," he says. "They remind us that there are others before us who suffered and were transformed. The world's great religious traditions offer exemplars of people who suffered— Moses, Jesus, Buddha, Mohammed. Their stories provide guidance and hope. They teach us that as bad as it feels now, suffering does not have to be the final word in life."

Buddhism, for example, is a religion steeped in ideas about suffering and enlightenment. It's clear in the religion's most basic story, about the Buddha's origin. The Buddha was the son of a king in northern India. His father wanted to protect him from all the evils of the world so he made sure that his son never left the palace grounds. He saw only young and beautiful servants. Anyone who was old or ill was removed. He never knew of the existence of poverty or suffering of any kind. He was even unaware of death.

After marrying the most beautiful woman in the land, he became restless and convinced a chariot driver to take him outside the palace grounds. There he saw an old man with wrinkles and gray hair. He was horrified and asked what was wrong with him and what he had done to deserve this. When the chariot driver explained that everyone gets old like this man, the Buddha was shocked and upset. He then saw a sick man, and then a dead man, and he was horrified to realize that people become ill and that everyone dies.

The young Buddha is traumatized by these revelations. He moves from living in a world free of illness, old age, and death to the realization that all of these terrible things will eventually befall him. At this point his world is turned upside down, says Daniel Veidlinger, an associate professor at California State University, Chico, who specializes in Eastern religions. Through this new knowledge, the young prince's entire worldview is shattered and he is overwhelmed with the prospect of a future that holds only suffering. What the Buddha suffers is in many ways the kind of seismic event that Tedeschi and Calhoun talk about, one that completely shakes the foundations of how an individual views the world.

But the story does not end with the trauma. Before his trip is over, the Buddha sees a fourth person, a holy man who has no possessions and is old but happy, living a simple life. The Buddha realizes that he wants to live like that. He dedicates his life to the pursuit of spiritual enlightenment. It is through suffering that Buddha is set on his path to enlightenment, perhaps the ultimate form of post-traumatic growth.

A transformation through suffering is also an important part of the Hindu epic, the Mahabharata, which tells, among other things, the story of five brothers who gamble their kingdom away to their cousins. After an exile of thirteen years during which they suffer greatly—they are attacked by wild animals and lose many friends and relatives—they return but are denied their kingdom. A bloody war ensues. Though the brothers ultimately win back their kingdom in battle, they are changed by the experience, says Veidlinger. "They are better people at the end of their thirteen years in exile than they were before; they are more aware of suffering in the world and they will never forget the terrible things that happened," he says. Untold numbers died in the battle to regain their kingdom and the rulers are haunted by those images for life. "They mournfully look back and remember the friends that were killed and they are better rulers because of it—more sensitive to others and to suffering," says Veidlinger.

Western religion has plenty to say about suffering, too. Jesus, of course, suffers terribly on the cross. And it is through his suffering that he is transformed, allowing him to rise to the kingdom of heaven. Paul Crowley, a theology professor at Santa Clara University and author of *Unwanted Wisdom: Suffering, the Cross, and Hope*, says that the image of the cross itself can become part of the psychological healing process. The cross, as a symbol of Jesus's suffering, forces Christians to confront their own traumatic experiences, their loss and grief and the suffering that ensues. And while avoiding memories and emotions associated with a traumatic event can be a helpful short-term means of coping with trauma, in the long term, confronting pain, suffering, and loss rather than avoiding it is a crucial step in healing from trauma. The symbol of the cross and the story behind it can provide hope, assuring the trauma survivor that he is not alone, that God also suffers and that he is surrounded by a community of those who suffer, says Crowley.

Even the story of Job from the Old Testament can provide some solace. In the story, Satan tells God that Job is faithful only because he has been rewarded with riches and a loving family. So God allows

Satan to afflict Job to prove the man's faith. Satan takes his children and his wealth. He tortures him with boils. Though Job argues with God, he does not renounce him. And in the end Job's family and riches are restored. It is a fairly bleak story with little redemption for Job. God does not explain much about what's behind his capricious cruelty, only pointing out that Job should not seek to understand God, the almighty creator of the universe. However, even this tale can provide some insight into the nature of trauma and suffering. "In one sense it tells us to just accept suffering as part of life with no rhyme or reason behind it," says Crowley. "But there is something more. Suffering also reveals some of the greater mystery of God."

While religious traditions have been helping people to understand trauma and loss for thousands of years, psychologists have long tiptoed around the question of the role that religion plays in healing from trauma. That may be because psychologists are much less religious than the general population and because religion does not fit neatly into much psychological research, says Pargament. He has spent his career looking at the question and has found that being religious can be helpful both when it comes to healing from trauma and when it comes to growth.

When religious people suffer a traumatic event, they are able to place their suffering in a larger context, he says. They can find some meaning in the experience and will be driven to search for significance in the event. "Faith can give their suffering a deeper meaning or purpose, another framework to explain their experience," he says.

Karanci, who has researched post-traumatic growth in Turkey, says that religion has been particularly helpful to earthquake survivors there. She has found that the survivors' faith helps them to accept the event that has led to the trauma because, from their perspective, the event comes from God. And they are quick to try to find meaning in the disaster, no matter how terrible. The trauma becomes like a cue for them to reassess their lives and try to lead better ones. "It is not a punishment for their sins," she says. "Instead it is like this event has a meaning and they've been leading a strange kind of life without really looking out for others and deeper relationships and so now they have to change."

The Struggle Is the Journey

Chery, like many religious people who suffer trauma, first felt betrayed by God. She had done everything the way she was supposed to. Yet her son still died. Her assumptive world, which included faith in the benevolence of God, was shattered. And so she first began to question her faith because it did not fit with the death of her son. "I don't think anyone is immune to this kind of struggle," says Pargament. "Their faith is shaken and that is okay; struggle is part of the spiritual journey." He points out that even Jesus on the cross struggled, asking why God has forsaken him. This struggle is one way that religious people handle trauma, something Pargament calls negative religious coping. And while it is often part of the process of coping with trauma for many religious people, those who do not move past it can face dire problems. Studies have shown that people who use only these negative coping styles have increased levels of distress, depression, anxiety, and post-traumatic stress symptoms.

But, Pargament says, for most people religious struggle is not the endpoint. It is only part of the process. They need to push back against their faith, to struggle with it in order to find a way to make peace with their trauma and their understanding of their religion and God. It is not unlike the process of accommodation in which the trauma survivor adapts his or her worldview to fit with the disruptive traumatic experience. William Feigelman, a retired professor of sociology at Nassau Community College in New York, has studied how religion helps the parents of children who have committed suicide. Many of the bereaved parents whom he spoke to during his research went through a period of alienation from God in much the way Chery did. But for most it didn't last. He says that those who were also able to find a sense of compassion and empathy were able to maintain and ultimately strengthen and deepen their faith.

Those who move on from their anger, hurt, and disappointment with their faith usually begin using what Pargament calls positive religious coping. It is an approach where survivors seek meaning from their experience, and hope and comfort from their beliefs, and gain some control over their reactions to the trauma, often with spiritual guidance. They then can find a new sense of closeness with God and others. Ultimately that process can lead to transformation or posttraumatic growth.

That process—the movement from trauma to anger and uncertainty to a search for meaning—is similar to what Tedeschi and Calhoun identified as well. The trauma has made the survivors' old way of understanding the world unworkable. They need to abandon it and find a new way of thinking about themselves, a new way of understanding the world around them. Those who view their lives and the trauma through a lens of religious faith will likely struggle with their understanding of their religion—their framework for understanding how the world works and how they should lead their lives. Then they will have to move forward, using deliberate rumination, narrative reframing, and other tools to build a new and often deeper sense of faith and spirituality.

It might seem that the less religious someone is, the easier this process might be. One's faith might be more malleable and less important, thereby making it easier to remold in a new and more relevant way. But that may not actually be the case. Feigelman studied 426 parents who had lost children to suicide. He discovered that the subjects who reported the most post-traumatic growth also reported the highest number of visits to church (the sample was predominantly Christian). "We were not surprised to find that the people who are more active churchgoers, who are more religious, score higher on these post-traumatic growth scales," he says. "Religion is a community anchorage. It gives someone something to hold on to when everything seems missing. People who lost a child enter into a state where everything is up for grabs and nothing makes sense. They have to make a new normal. Bereaved people have to do this, they have to make new meaning."

A number of subsequent studies have found a high correlation between religious faith and growth. One study published in 2006 assessed two groups of breast cancer survivors five and eight years after their surgery. Researchers found that those who reported the most positive changes also reported that they used religion as a way of coping with their cancer. One large review of 103 studies of post-traumatic growth found that religious coping was more often correlated with growth than most other attributes, including community support or optimism—though those were not too far behind. For many, religious faith is a key to finding meaning in traumatic suffering.

Many Faiths Can Offer a Path to Growth

As Chery began to engage again with her priest and with friends, she also educated herself about what she had been through. She learned about PTSD, and once she had a name for the reaction she was having to the loss of her son, she felt empowered. And soon she began searching for what else might come from this trauma. "Once I knew that bad things could happen to me I wanted to figure out, what are the good things that can happen to me?" she says. She read self-help books like Rick Warren's *The Purpose Driven Life* and Deepak Chopra's *The Seven Spiritual Laws of Success*. She had never been much of a reader but now, after her son's death, she forced herself to read at least a chapter a day. Then she tried to apply what she was reading to her daily life. "You had to make the conscious decision, do I want to be in chaos and confusion and calamity or do I want to be in comfort and peace and unity?" she says. Chery decided to pursue the latter and to try to bring something positive into the world for herself and her children. She felt it was her duty to herself and to God. She asked herself again and again, How can I be the person that God has called me to be?

Chery began to think about her son's goals in life and what she might be able to do to honor him, to lead her life in a way that would be a tribute to him. She worked with the Boston public school system to develop a curriculum around Louis that discusses his life and death and includes reading some of the books he loved. And she founded the Louis D. Brown Peace Institute, which provides help and services to family members who have lost a child to gun violence. She speaks regularly about Louis and her work promoting peace in cities and curbing gun violence. "I need to be able to find a way to use my grief and pain, what I have gone through, to channel that into something positive and at the same time to help other survivors to mentor those who are going through this," she says. The tagline to her organization: "Transforming pain and anger into power and action." That is exactly what she has managed to do and it's a path she wants to help other grieving parents to discover, too.

Despite all she is doing to help others, Chery is still in pain. She still misses her son terribly. She continues to rely on friends and family for help. "I surround myself with people who are going to allow me to go through my grief and trauma, my rage and anger, and who are going to pull me up when I need to be pulled up," she says. "I have a good safe space where I can dump the stuff that I am dealing with, and not carry it all the time. And when I release it I am much lighter." Prayer and her relationship with God have played a central role in that, too. She prays daily and pledges to make her thoughts and action one and the same.

Chery's faith is different than it was before Louis died, says her oldest sister, Julia Thompson. "The depth of her faith is very profound," she says. "I think she is more in tune with her reason to be on this earth. I think she believes there is a purpose as to why this happened to her child and to her, that God has a plan for her." Chery says that she sees her faith as a lifelong journey towards inner peace. She now lives her life according to seven guiding principles: love, unity, faith, hope, courage, justice, and forgiveness. "I mindfully make the choice to use the principles as my strategy to receive and share God's gift of peace," she says. And she is only here today because of her faith. "Louis's death, painful as it is, I know that it is not something that God willed, but by the grace of God I am here twenty years later," she says. Without her faith and the church she could never do what she is doing. "I would be addicted to drugs, I would want to forget about it, I would be a very bitter woman. I am angry, but instead of the anger destroying me, I learned to control the anger rather than letting it control me," she says. "I thank God for pulling me up and I pray that I serve him in the way he wants me to serve him."

While Chery is a Christian, it is not only Christianity than can help trauma survivors. Other religions can be helpful in surprisingly similar ways, says Avinash Thombre, an associate professor in the department of speech communication at the University of Arkansas at Little Rock. Because most of the research on the role of religion in trauma recovery has been conducted in the United States, Thombre, who is from India, wanted to know more about how religion helped to inform the lives of cancer survivors there.

For a 2010 study, he and a group of colleagues surveyed and interviewed sixty-one breast cancer patients. Nearly all the subjects were Hindu and the important role religion played in their lives was clear from the start. As part of their religion, Hindus believe that this life is just one of many they have lived and will live. That concept, combined with the idea of karma—that one's actions in previous lives impact the future—helped to frame their understanding of their cancer diagnosis. Hindus often believe that when bad things befall them, it is because of something bad that they did in a previous life. Many of the cancer patients began by thinking they got cancer because of bad karma, and that helped them to accept the illness. In addition, most of the women also felt obligated to fight the cancer. God wanted them to fight it for their children and families. They felt obligated by their religious beliefs to get better. "It was their spirituality, religion, and family obligations that gave them strength," Thombre says.

He also found that the women became much more engaged spiritually as they went through their treatment. "They went back to the temple and they were praying together. They were not seeking out the guru or the temple priest; they were just being more spiritual," he says. "They really spent time there chanting and taking part in the acts."

Being engaged spiritually, Thombre says, helped them to transform their understanding of themselves. They started out as victims of the cancer but quickly viewed themselves instead as fighters and survivors. "It crystallized that idea even more that you are a fighter, that you want to do this for your family," he says. And that helped them to see their own inner strength.

Thombre and his colleagues conducted another study in India of fifty-eight caregivers of cancer patients. This group used many of the same approaches that Pargament outlined in his work. Many struggled to reconcile their loved one's cancer with their idea of a benevolent God—negative religious coping. And Thombre found that many eventually found a path to a more positive means of religious coping. That positive coping was highly correlated with growth in exactly the same way that Pargament found it was with Christians in the United States. The cultural and religious settings could not be more different, but the mechanisms that allowed faith to spur growth remained the same.

Pargament is convinced that the particulars of faith and even spirituality are less important than some of the underlying similarities. In fact, he has begun trying to use some of the same mechanisms that he sees working in religious people with those who are not particularly religious at all. Anyone's recovery can be aided by discovering things in their lives that are sacred, he says. Tapping into one's sense of the sacred can help to activate some of those processes that are so helpful to religious trauma survivors. Chery, for example, felt that God had called her to help others after her son's death and so she founded the Louis D. Brown Peace Institute. The work she does there is sacred—it is infused with a deeper meaning because of its connection to her son. Similarly, most people have something in their lives that they consider sacred regardless of their faith. If they can identify those things that have the deepest meaning and then work to better incorporate them into their lives, they are more likely to heal from trauma and change for the better, says Pargament. "It can be anything, a loving relationship, work, the environment, making the world a better place," he says. "I am helping trauma victims find new sources of sacred meaning and value."

With these sacred pursuits as a guide, people can reorient their lives, find meaningful goals, and ultimately grow. "With people who are depressed, who have experienced PTSD, who have lost everything, I ask them to dig down deep, to find what makes them special, what lights them up, where the spark is," Pargament says. "And I ask them to fan that spark into a flame and when they do, amazing things happen."

CHAPTER 9

Opening Up to New Experiences

Creativity Spurs Change

STANDING OFF TO THE SIDE OF THE PEDESTRIAN WALKWAY THAT runs over the Brooklyn Bridge, Bob Carey removed a small pink tutu from his backpack. Bending over, he pulled the tutu over his bare feet and up over his baggy khaki shorts. Then he dropped his shorts.

"Look at my butt," Carey said to a friend. "Are my shorts showing?" He meant the pink shorts that he wore beneath the tutu so he wouldn't get arrested for indecent exposure. None was visible. He took off his T-shirt and then walked to a spot on the path right on the dividing line between the pedestrian walkway and the bicycle lane. Carey, who is fifty-three and not exactly model-thin or model-hairless, turned his back to his camera, which he had mounted on a tripod in the middle of the walkway. He bowed his head and extended his arms down and outward from his body so they hovered above the pink fringe of the tutu. With a tiny black clicker—a remote control for the camera—in his hand, he began to take photo after photo of himself posed on the walkway as bicyclists zipped past and pedestrians lingered to look at the view. One of the bridge's iconic stone towers loomed above him and the Brooklyn skyline took on an orange glow in the distance as the sun set behind him over Manhattan.

As he clicked away, a crowd of tourists and locals began to gather, watching him standing in the middle of the bridge in nothing but his tutu. In just a minute or two Carey was satisfied that he got what he needed.

"What's this for?" asked one woman in the crowd as Carey made his way back to his camera, where the group was assembled.

"I've been doing this for ten years all around the world to raise money for breast cancer patients," Carey told the group. "My wife has had cancer for ten years."

Carey reached into his bag, still wearing just his tutu, and pulled out stickers and postcards and began handing them out to the people in the crowd around him.

"Oh, okay," said the woman. "That puts a whole different spin on things. Now it makes sense."

"Here you go," said Carey as he handed out more stickers and postcards. "We raise money, we sell books," he said.

Carey's wife, Linda Lancaster-Carey, was diagnosed with breast cancer in 2003. The cancer recurred in her liver in 2006, and she has been in treatment ever since. Carey, a commercial and fine art photographer, has been taking pictures of himself in that pink tutu for a decade. When his wife started chemotherapy after her cancer returned in 2006, she took the photos with her on her iPad to help pass the time during appointments. Soon she started showing them to other women in chemotherapy with her. They loved them. Carey was shooting himself in all kinds of environments: the bustle of Times Square, the wide-open and empty spaces of Monument Valley, leaping into the water off Martha's Vineyard, asleep in a New

Jersey hotel room. The images are funny, sad, whimsical, thought-provoking, and totally engaging. She encouraged him to shoot more of them.

In 2012, they self-published a book of the images. When they posted images on Facebook, there was an overwhelming response. Executives at Deutsche Telekom, the German telecommunications firm, took notice. They flew Carey and his wife to Germany, filmed a commercial with them, sponsored a gallery show of his work, and spent millions airing the ad. They have been on the *Today* show and are now also sponsored by Bloomingdale's. They have sold out of their book and have raised more than two hundred thousand dollars for their foundation, which distributes funds to other organizations that help cancer patients pay for costs like transportation to doctor's appointments, wigs, and child care that are not covered by insurance.

"I can't believe that is the man," said a woman on the bridge in a German accent to her two friends as Carey handed out stickers and cards. "Can we have a photo with you?" she asked. "We have seen you on TV."

Carey posed with the women and the man while another onlooker snapped the photo.

"He's very famous," the woman said to the impromptu photographer.

"Bye-bye, have a safe journey home," said Carey to the trio as they left. "We love Germany. We might be back in September. We will see you."

And with that the crowd slowly dispersed. Carey took off the tutu and put his shorts on, gathered his equipment, and, with a friend who helped him with the shoot, started walking back toward Brooklyn, where his car was parked.

• • •

Lancaster-Carey grew up in Michigan. She was the eighth of nine children and, according to her sister, Lori Lancaster, she was always drawn to art. "She was always strong and independent and a free-thinker," she says. "Linda was very creative." Lancaster-Carey says that with so many siblings she was largely left to figure things out on her own. "When there's nine kids, it's sort of hard not to be independent. Someone had to take care of me and it was me," she says.

In her early twenties Lancaster-Carey moved to Phoenix, Arizona, to go to school for graphic design. A few years later she met Carey, who was a working photographer at the time. "I remember our first real date. We were sitting at a light and we'd have been in the car for like two miles and we're laughing at something really stupid, but it was funny to us," she says. "I thought, Oh my gosh, I haven't made sense for the last two miles and this guy thinks I'm funny. This is good."

Soon Lancaster-Carey found herself working with Carey. He needed help setting up his business, and she knew a number of photographers that she could ask for advice. With Lancaster-Carey managing the business, Carey had more time to focus on the creative work and the couple built a flourishing commercial photography business.

At the same time Carey pursued long-term art projects, too. Over the course of a decade he took images of himself with his head and face shaved clean and painted silver, others of his head wrapped tightly in fishing wire to distort his features. "I started in 1993 because I was stressed by personal problems and I would wrap my head up in a fishing line," says Carey. "These self-portraits, for over twenty years, have always just been about taking care of myself. It's my self-therapy and self-healing."

But after twenty years in Phoenix, Carey was itching for something new and challenging. He wanted to move to New York. They both had friends in the city and one of Lancaster-Carey's sisters lived there. So in the spring of 2003 they sold off what they could and packed the rest of their belongings into a rental truck and set out for New York.

On the first day of their trip, they stopped to visit friends in Santa Fe. They had a barn on their property and something about that view got Carey thinking. He ran to the back of the truck and pulled out a pink tutu packed in one of the boxes. It was a leftover from an earlier project he had done for Ballet Arizona. He put it on and stood in front of the barn in his white socks and the pink-fringed skirt and snapped some images. Then the couple went back on their way. He wasn't sure what to do with the photograph. That summer he took a few more images of himself in the tutu but he still wasn't sure where the ideas was going.

Relocating to New York was more challenging than they expected. Work came in slowly and Carey wasn't sure if they were going to make it. He even thought that maybe he'd have to give up photography entirely and try to get a job—doing what, he couldn't imagine.

And then, eight months after they arrived in New York, Lancaster-Carey found a lump in her breast. She had an appointment for a mammogram on Christmas Eve. Carey's grandfather had just passed away and so he had had to leave town. Lancaster-Carey felt that she was fine on her own and told Carey not to worry about coming back early. When the test results were in, the doctor called her into his office. "I can still hear the paper crinkle as I'm sitting there dangling my legs," says Lancaster-Carey. "She said, 'I'm really sorry but you have cancer.' My mind went numb. And I'm thinking, I can't call anybody. Everybody I know is out of town." When Carey came back from his trip, she told him the news.

Lancaster-Carey's tumor was formed like a web and was growing inward, making it impossible for doctors to even get a clear image of it. Lancaster-Carey was only forty-three when she was diagnosed and she wasn't ready to face the possibility of such an illness, the disfiguration that the surgery would cause, and the possibility of death. Cancer was pervasive in their lives. Lancaster-Carey's grandmother and uncle had died from cancer, and Carey's mother and godmother had died of breast cancer, and his sister was diagnosed with it a month after his wife was. "I was young and that was huge to have to think about something like that. Not that there was another option. There was no option," she says.

But at the same time, Lancaster-Carey felt like she had ways of handling adversity. "I had done a lot of meditation, Reiki, a lot of art therapy, dance therapy, getting your emotions out through your writing, your drawing. I already had what I call my bag of tricks," she says. "All of these years I was doing all of this stuff and this was just waiting for me. I thought I was very fortunate."

Lancaster-Carey was in surgery a long time. The cancer had spread to her lymph nodes. She stayed in the hospital recovering for four days. Despite the support from her friends and family, when she was released she was afraid of what the future might hold. But she quickly turned to her bag of tricks—therapies and creative means of expression—to help her confront those feelings and find a path forward.

Lancaster-Carey wrote in her journal. And she drew. "They were quick drawings, there wasn't any art involved. It was just to get my feelings out. It could have been pastels. I use a lot of pastels. It was more the color that showed my emotion than whatever I was drawing. They weren't great works of art," she says. "It just helped me to deal with it. I was just talking to myself." She also remembered the dance therapy class she took years earlier. In the class the instructor would choose the music and guide students through a dance, giving them something to think about. Then the students would move their bodies as a way of responding to their thoughts and emotions. "After the surgery, I wasn't doing a whole lot of moving but at least it gave me creative ways to find an outlet," says Lancaster-Carey. "It really helped."

After six months of chemotherapy and thirty-three radiation treatments, Lancaster-Carey was accepted into a clinical trial that lasted for another year. Through all of that, Carey was taking pictures of himself in the tutu. "It was really hard to talk to him about this," she says. "We watched his mom die of breast cancer, so automatically you know what can happen, and then you hear your wife has one of the most aggressive forms of cancer and you have no work and I'm sure it messed his mind up. I saw emotionally what that was doing to him. I'd bring home pamphlets for support groups but he just wasn't interested in that. He went to counseling on his own and then with friends. And then, ironically the tutu started helping out."

Creativity Drives Growth

For both Lancaster-Carey and her husband, art worked as therapy to help them get through the struggles each of them faced in the wake of the cancer diagnosis, the treatments, the loss of family members, and the cold possibility of death that suddenly entered their lives. Art therapy has long been used to help people with a range of problems, from survival of adverse events to struggles with illness, both physical and mental.

Adrian Hill is credited with first using art as a tool for helping those in physical and mental distress. He was a British government war artist on the Western Front in World War I and accompanied soldiers in battle to sketch and paint battlefield scenes. While recovering from tuberculosis, he realized how helpful his art was in his own recovery process. He began teaching art to others at the facility, many of whom were fellow veterans suffering from physical injuries and shell shock. He was impressed with how drawing and painting seemed to help them. Others took up the practice in Europe and the United States, and in the 1950s and 1960s art therapy grew in popularity and acceptance.

Today art therapy is well established and encompasses a broad range of approaches. Expressive writing, discussed earlier, is considered one form of art therapy, so is the use of visual arts such as painting and sculpture, as well as performance arts such as music and dance—any means of creative expression that has therapeutic value for those suffering from post-traumatic stress and a host of other problems is considered a form of art therapy. Some approaches to art therapy have resulted in improved physical health, reducing the length of hospital stays for those suffering from illness, for example. Other studies show that art therapy can boost quality of life and decrease depression and anxiety in cancer patients. For many, this form of expression is a powerful tool for coping with the psychological struggles that come from surviving trauma.

Those who use these therapies with their patients say that it works because it helps focus people on new activities that absorb them in the process of creating something. That absorption, or flow, an intense concentration that merges both action and awareness, has benefits. It can produce a sense of competence and accomplishment, and positive emotion. People enjoy it and engaging in an enjoyable activity has its own benefits, particularly as one struggles with deep and sometimes overwhelming problems. And tapping into creative ways of thinking in art can help inspire people to find more creative ways to address their problems.

For Carey, creating his series of self-portraits provided him with the time he needed for himself, to explore his emotions, his fear and love and the changes this illness brought to his relationship. "One of the reasons why I do what I do is that [the possibility of Lancaster-Carey's death] scares the hell out of me," Carey says. "I can't imagine going through that." And, says Lancaster-Carey, the project allowed her husband to find the refuge that he needed in his art. Carey would take day trips, or Lancaster-Carey would come along with him. He would never leave unless she was feeling healthy enough to come along or be on her own. "It was also a way for him to leave, and I've always recognized that, that he needed to do his own artwork," she says. "That's what he needs to do, to explore his life through his art."

In 2006, after doctors found cancer in her liver, Lancaster-Carey began sharing the images with the other women she met at her chemotherapy treatments. "We would laugh. They loved it. They thought it was funny. Some of them saw the art in it. Some of them saw the humor. Some of them saw the melancholy," she says. And that was a nice feeling, to share something that she and Carey had worked on, to get that kind of reaction from people who were going through the same turmoil that she was.

The more people reacted to the images, the more Lancaster-Carey started thinking about a conversation she had in a support group early in her cancer. "People were asking me, 'What are you going to do with your life now that you've had cancer?'" she says. The question bothered her. What did they mean? "My response was, 'I am going to live my life. Am I supposed to be doing something bigger than what I'm doing now?' And if I was in a touchy mood, I'd think, What, I am not living my life big enough just by living it?" she says.

But something about that question gnawed at her. "I had asked myself that question someplace way back here," she said, gesturing to the back of her head. "Maybe I could make a difference somehow. The seed was there and hopefully I'd notice it when it knocks on my door." And when she realized how much other people were connecting with her husband's self-portraits, she knew that she had found what she was looking for. The Tutu Project was knocking.

In 2008 the couple wrote a book proposal. The idea was to publish a book, sell it, and distribute it to cancer centers to raise awareness and money for those undergoing treatment. They got an agent. Publishers were interested. Then the economy crashed in 2008 and the one publisher who had been sitting on the proposal for eight months suddenly turned it down. Shortly afterward Carey's father died, and Lancaster-Carey lost a brother-in-law, both to cancer. When the couple returned from the funerals they loaded their dogs into a van and set out on a ten-day road trip to shoot more images. It was the only way the two of them could deal with the death and bad news invading every corner of their lives.

On the last day of their trip, they were shooting in Wildwood, New Jersey, a tourist town on the shore. They were too tired to make it all the way back to Brooklyn, so they drove around late at night looking for a place to stay. It was the off-season, and their only option was a run-down motel. When they opened the door, however, they knew they had gotten very lucky. Sure, the carpet was so gross that Lancaster-Carey kept her shoes on all night. But hanging above one of the twin beds was a paint-by-numbers picture of a ballerina. They moved the picture so it hung between the beds and then got to work setting up a shot. The pair worked until 2 a.m. on getting the image of Carey in his tutu, lying on one of the beds, half out of the frame, curled up and asleep, just right. "I remember saying, 'Would you shoot this already? I want to go to bed,'" says Lancaster-Carey.

"When I look at the image, I see all this emotion and I'm hearing in my head, It's two o'clock in the morning and I want to go to bed."

Frustrated with the lack of interest, they shelved the project for a while. But later, when they showed the work from the trip, including that hotel image, to a friend, they got excited about their idea again. Their friend thought the images were fantastic and he pushed them to take another shot at publishing a book. The couple decided they would just do it themselves. They spent a year working on it together and paid for the project out of their own pocket. They called it *Ballerina*.

When they started posting images on Facebook to promote the book, and explained their goal of raising money to help cancer patients, people responded. Images were getting thousands of likes from people. The couple was invited to shoot an image with the American Ballet Theatre. Deutsche Telekom flew them to Germany, where crowds of cancer survivors turned up to meet them, to hug them and cry. It was overwhelming but also moving and very satisfying.

But Carey isn't tempted to cater the work to his growing audience. His art remains his art, no matter how much it moves other people. "I've never tried to please people with these," he says. "It's always been about my sensibility. I'm not going, 'Oh my God, people are going to love this one.' It's just for me." And it has to remain something he does for himself. "I just think about making photographs and meeting people and having little adventures in the middle of nowhere and to not think about reality, maybe. And that's what I think I was doing when Linda was sick."

Lancaster-Carey's sister, Lori Lancaster, isn't surprised that the project arose from her sister's cancer. "The way she thinks is, Okay, so I have this, what can I create from this experience?" Lancaster-Carey says there have been other changes to her life, too. "There was a panel of women at St. Vincent's [Hospital, in New York City] and this one woman said cancer was the best thing that ever happened to her. And I'm thinking in my head, Are you out of your mind? How could this possibly be? I would never say that, but yes, I have changed. I didn't get caught up with what people thought of me too much before, but now I just don't care. If there is a challenge, I'm thinking, I have cancer, how hard can it be? Or if there is a problem with the business, it's like, Okay, but I'm still alive. So my perspective has changed. It has furthered my growth," she says. "It has probably made me a lot stronger. I drive Bob crazy because I don't get caught up in a lot of stuff with other people or business. I don't have time for games."

Openness to New Experiences Helps Spur Change

Linda Lancaster-Carey and Bob Carey are creative people. Making art is at the core of how they reflect, engage, and understand who they are and how the world works. Art is at the core of their post-traumatic growth. And that is no surprise.

One of the personality traits often correlated with post-traumatic growth is openness to new experience. People who have this trait often have an interest in, and appreciation for, art. They are more emotional, adventurous, imaginative, and curious. They are willing to try new things. And openness to new experience is the personality trait most predictive of creativity.

In a way, post-traumatic growth almost requires a certain amount of creativity. One must think creatively about one's life, one's past, and the possibilities for the future, in order to grow. It is a creative leap. That process of deliberate rumination that Tedeschi and Calhoun describe is, at its core, a creative process, one of considering, understanding, reimagining. "Expressing yourself in one form or another is important in terms of the process of adapting to trauma and achieving some sense of growth," says Queensland University of Technology's Jane Shakespeare-Finch. And while she says any means of expression—simply writing or talking—can be effective, she adds, "Creative people have more doorways to expressing themselves than those who are not creative."

In 1989, Tobi Zausner, a New York artist, was diagnosed with aggressive ovarian cancer. She had surgery. Given the size of the tumor and speed with which it had grown, her doctor didn't expect her to live more than two or three months. She was overcome by bouts of nausea and severe vomiting. "It was awful," says Zausner. She practiced meditation, and Chinese exercises called Soaring Crane Qigong. She improved her diet and read books about those who survived cancer and in time she, too, healed and survived.

At the time of her diagnosis, Zausner was pursuing a degree in psychology but had not finished her dissertation. Afterward, she went on to complete a Ph.D. in art and psychology and became a licensed clinical social worker with a private practice. "I became a research psychologist. I never expected to do that," she says. Zausner also wrote a book about illness and creativity called *When Walls Become Doorways: Creativity and the Transforming Illness*, which chronicles not only her story but those of dozens of artists and creative people who have found new meaning and new direction in their lives and in their art after calamities. For her and those she has written about, adversity, even the most severe kind—paralysis, terminal illness, and others—is a catalyst for new ways of seeing, understanding, and creating, pushing artists to reinvent themselves and their work. "For creative people it is like a reflex action, to turn traumatic experience into creative work," says Zausner. "We transmogrify the pain into creative output. In just doing that there is an enormous feeling of centering.

It's very calming, very focusing, very strengthening. Making the work becomes therapeutic."

Zausner's book is filled with dozens of examples of artists, some famous and some less known, who survived terrible experiences, only to have those events either change their lives, their art, or both.

Henri Matisse, she points out, had no interest in art until he was twenty years old. Through his entire life he had chronic digestive problems. He was deemed too sickly to take over his father's business, which was passed on to his younger brother, marking him as a failure. He became a law clerk, but he hated the work. When he lived in Paris for a year as a law student, he never once visited the Louvre Museum.

When he was twenty he had an acute problem with his intestines, resulting in severe and debilitating pain. With no cure available, he was ordered to rest until the pain subsided. While in the hospital, he noticed that the man next to him was using a type of early paint-by-numbers set called chromos. Matisse was intrigued. He asked his mother for a set and was hooked. "The moment I had this box of colors in my hands, I had the feeling that my life was there," he wrote. After he was released from the hospital, he was set on a totally different trajectory. He eventually quit the law office and left for Paris to pursue his career as an artist.

Matisse would have several more severe illnesses in his life. When he was in his early seventies he underwent surgery for intestinal cancer. The cancer and complications from the surgery—pulmonary embolisms, a prolapsed stomach, and the flu—left him wheelchair-bound for the rest of his life. But he refused to stop making art. Before he could get out of bed, he used a fishing rod with charcoal on the end to draw on the walls and ceiling. When he could sit up and later use a wheelchair, he started making colorful cutouts that were assembled on the wall by his assistants. Zausner says that these forms moved for Matisse when he no longer could. And, she says, they are among his best work (a 2014 exhibit of the cutouts broke attendance records at the Tate Modern museum in London). Matisse struggled later with gallstones and other complications. Doctors didn't expect him to live. But Matisse found new meaning in both his life and his work after the surgery. "Only what I created after my illness constitutes my real self," he told an interviewer.

"He had such enormous post-traumatic growth after each of these difficult illnesses," says Zausner. "For him creativity was so healing." Through plumbing the lives of artists past and present, Zausner has found deep anecdotal links between creative people and their ability to grow from their traumatic experiences. "It's like a singularity in physics that you go through and you just reorganize on the other side. You can reorganize any way you want to," says Zausner. "And for some people suffering turns into growth."

Can Trauma Spur Creativity?

Matisse and these other artists were able to grow from their experiences in part because of their creative approach to life and their work. But Zausner also argues that the trauma actually pushed the artists such as Matisse to new heights—the trauma made them better artists. And from a psychologist's point of view, that shift in artistic output can be a kind of growth. Marie Forgeard, a doctoral candidate studying at the Positive Psychology Center at the University of Pennsylvania, was intrigued by the relationship between trauma and art. Adverse events, even horrible traumas, are remarkably common in the lives of celebrated artists. Maya Angelou, for example, was raped by her mother's boyfriend when she was eight years old. Frida Kahlo survived polio, a terrible traffic accident, and three miscarriages. Film director Francis

Ford Coppola also had polio as a child. One study found that writers were more likely than others in the general population to be orphaned.

Forgeard wanted to examine whether adverse experiences or traumatic events boosted the creativity of her subjects—something she calls creative growth. To do so, she asked 373 people to describe how the most difficult experience of their lives affected them. She found that those who reported positive changes in their interpersonal relationships and increased perception of new possibilities (two of the five areas of growth defined by Tedeschi and Calhoun) also reported enhanced creativity—growth in these areas and creativity seemed to be increasing together.

Yet those who experienced positive changes were not the only ones who reported an increase in creativity. Subjects in the study who reported negative changes in interpersonal relationships also reported enhanced creativity, indicating that the struggle with adversity may also push people creatively. Some people may be using their creative skills to work through their traumatic experiences and finding that the struggle with that experience boosts creativity, too.

And it turns out that those who are predisposed to creativity may be more likely than others to experience creative growth. Many creative people are necessarily introspective. They absorb, they think, they try to understand their experience, often through their own creative process. Artists are often well versed in deliberate rumination, the cognitive process that Tedeschi and Calhoun say helps many people find a path to post-traumatic growth. In a separate study, Forgeard found that those subjects who experienced high levels of adversity and scored high on openness to new experience, a personality trait that is related to creativity, reported more creative growth than others in the study. "The higher people were in openness to new experience, the more creative growth they reported," says Forgeard.

For Lancaster-Carey and her husband, their creative approach to life, their training and work as artists, the way they view the world, their place in it, and their possibilities all certainly contributed to the growth that they both experienced. And it allowed them to find a way to use those skills to heal themselves and heal others.

Lancaster-Carey and her husband eventually left Brooklyn. The borough had become too expensive. They packed up and moved to a small house in Saddle River, New Jersey, on a quiet, almost rural street. Carey has a studio in the basement. On the main floor, their dog, Sofie, has the run of the place and barks at the slightest squeak in the old cottage.

Carey is gruff and funny and not one to sentimentalize. He talks critically about himself, his motives, and his work, as if the entire enterprise might fall apart if he were to relax and enjoy the good press and the success the couple has earned with the Tutu Project. But Lancaster-Carey's sister says that the project affected Carey in ways he rarely discusses. "The Tutu Project is his saving grace," says Lancaster. "He is willing to share everything. As an artist he has put everything into his work. It has also touched him knowing that he is helping other people as well as his wife." The fact that the images have so much reach now, that they have helped so many people, that the couple is able to raise money to give to those who need it, is very meaningful to Carey and has helped him to see his art in a new light.

Sitting at his dining room table in a paint-splotched black T-shirt, with Lancaster-Carey at his side, he says, "I think this is probably the most important thing I'll ever do because it has impacted so many people. That it has helped other people, I never imagined that at all. Ever."

PART THREE

Cultivating Growth

Putting the Tools for Growth to Use

CHAPTER 10

Racing Boats and Climbing Mountains

Getting Active Opens the Door to Growth

EARLY ON A SATURDAY MORNING IN SEPTEMBER TWENTY WOMEN sat in two long and perilously narrow boats tied to a dock in Flushing Bay in Queens, New York. Wearing baseball hats, sunglasses, and life jackets and clutching paddles, they listened to one of their coaches, Akila Simon, as she got them fired up for the morning workout.

"Close the door on fear as you paddle today. If you are afraid to get down close to the water today, let that fear out and go for it. You are superstrong," she told the women. "Throw fear out the window."

And with that the women pushed the boats back from the dock, turned them, and paddled out into the bay, where the tip of LaGuardia Airport's runway meets the water.

Donna Wilson, a cofounder of this group, the Empire Dragon Boat Team, stood at the back of one of the boats holding a long paddle that is used like a rudder to steer. As the women paddled, launching the boat forward with each stroke, practicing starts and sprints, Wilson shouted at them encouragingly, but also a little intimidatingly. "Dig it, dig it down!" she yelled, urging the women to get their paddles deep into the water so they would get more power on each stroke.

For nearly two hours that morning, the women zipped back and forth across the bay in their long, narrow dragon boats, a type of boat that is traditionally raced in China. They raced each other in short, all-out sprints and longer, paced distances. During short breaks, women yelled good-natured put-downs across the water at each other to inspire the competition.

These women are serious competitors, but they are not just any group of rowers. This dragon boat team is part of an international league of boats raced entirely by breast cancer survivors. Wilson, who helped start the team, is a nurse and personal trainer at Memorial Sloan Kettering Cancer Center in New York City. When she came to the hospital in 1992, she was working with lung cancer patients, and she discovered that if patients exercised for just three weeks prior to surgery, they had much better outcomes. She knew from both research and her firsthand observations that exercise was important for recovery, too, but others seemed unaware of the value of staying active. Doctors and nurses routinely told cancer patients to just rest after chemotherapy, without mentioning the value of fitness. After such a long stretch of inactivity, it took most cancer survivors a year of hard work to get back into reasonable shape following remission.

When Wilson began working with breast cancer patients, the situation was even worse. After surgery, women were told that they couldn't lift more than five pounds and couldn't do upper-body exercises involving repetitive motion. Doctors feared that it would increase the possibility of lymphedema, a common complication for breast cancer survivors that causes painful swelling of the arms. But there was little research to back up this assumption. Finally, in 2009, the first long-term study of the effects of upper-body exercise in breast cancer survivors was published. It showed that there was no link between the workouts and lymphedema.

While researching potential exercise programs for breast cancer survivors, Wilson found a study that revealed significant benefits from dragon boat racing. She'd never heard of dragon boats before, but she quickly discovered that the sport had been growing for years—the first dragon boat team comprised of breast cancer survivors was founded in 1996 and today there are more than 110 teams around the world. It seemed like a great way to get women exercising and keep them active and engaged with their health and fitness. When Wilson started her team in 2009, doctors at Memorial Sloan Kettering were skeptical. "I had some people saying you can't do this," says Wilson. But the team's success has helped to overcome that skepticism. "Now I feel so proud to watch the passion in these women that never really exercised before, to see them get fit, watch their diet. They are totally different women," says Wilson. "It is very exciting to see the change in them."

In one of the dragon boats out on Flushing Bay that morning, Heather Maloney plunged her paddle into the water and pulled back with her whole body, tensing the muscles in her shoulder and neck. She kept her head looking forward and her arms straight, focused on keeping time with the woman paddling in front of her as Wilson shouted at the rowers. Maloney, who today is trim and fit with short blond hair peeking out from beneath her cap, was diagnosed with breast cancer in 2009, when she was forty-four. Cancer was something she was quite familiar with—at the time she was the executive director of a pediatric cancer organization and spent a lot of her time in cancer wards. But nothing prepared her for the way cancer would upend her own life. The day after her diagnosis, she began making changes.

"I woke up the next day knowing a few things and one was that I wasn't going to die in this apartment on East Seventy-Eighth Street," she says of her home at the time. She quickly moved to a tiny waterfront community on the New Jersey side of the Hudson River. Now she wakes up to birds in the morning instead of delivery trucks. She also decided that she would forgive everyone in advance for all of the insensitive and inappropriate things they were going to say to her (thanks to her job, she knew that even the most well-meaning friends and relatives can say rude and insensitive things out of sheer fear and awkwardness). And she would accept everything and anything that people gave her—time, food, clothes, money—without guilt. "I never questioned myself," says Maloney. "There is such freedom when death is possible, you become very present in your life in a way that is different. All the BS flies out the window."

Maloney's treatments were brutal. Her surgeon removed thirteen lymph nodes—three tested positive for cancer. She endured six months of chemotherapy and participated in a clinical trial as well. "It was like being in a vat of chemicals. It was a horrible drug," she says. She had thirty radiation treatments. An expander, an inflatable implant, was placed under the muscles in her chest to stretch them out to make room for a permanent implant. It stayed there for eight months and was incredibly painful. Then came hormone therapy—she's halfway through a ten-year protocol. "The fatigue was bone crushing," she says. "I had joint pain. It was like being old. I wondered if I would ever feel well again."

Maloney had never played sports growing up and never considered herself particularly athletic. But when she heard about the dragon boat team at the hospital, it sounded appealing. Maloney isn't married and has no children. Hobbies and groups are important to her. The idea of being part of a team sounded right. "The moment I sliced a paddle in the water, I knew. I knew immediately I was in," she says.

The team is a serious commitment. The women go through dry-land training in the off-season. They are on the water twice a week, in Flushing Bay, which is better known for dead rats, floating garbage, and sewage overflow than as the venue for any serious athletic endeavor. Team members are rarely permitted to miss practice, so summer vacations are curtailed. The commitment and the competitive focus appealed to Maloney.

Not long after she joined, she found another, less obvious benefit. The team is its own remarkable community. Every year the group takes a trip to Florida for early-season training. The women stay together, train together all day, every day. Their friendships deepen and they come together as a team. In the off-season they do volunteer work together. They have all become good friends, bonding over their sport and also their common cancer experience. They make light of their fears—every ache and pain is an indication of a new cancer about to spring on them. "We have this ability to talk about our experiences with people who understand. There is a humor to it that we couldn't have with our [other] friends. They would be horrified," Maloney says.

It is just that kind of social connection that has been so helpful to these women. As one researcher found, it's likely the secret ingredient that helps these cancer survivors to grow.

Meghan McDonough, an associate professor in the department of health and kinesiology at Purdue University, had been a competitive paddler since high school and had raced dragon boats and coached paddlers since 2001. She was curious about how the sport was benefiting breast cancer survivors. For a study published in 2007, McDonough and her colleagues interviewed twenty breast cancer survivors on a dragon boat team in Vancouver, British Columbia. It was the kind of qualitative study that Tedeschi and Calhoun had used decades earlier, simply asking broad questions and recording the answers. McDonough found widespread post-traumatic growth among the twenty women they interviewed. Seventy-five percent of them reported having closer personal relationships and indicated that they were pursuing new possibilities in their lives. Almost 90 percent of them reported that they felt stronger as a result of the program. And 65 percent reported an increased appreciation for life. Though this is a tiny sample, the results indicate that these breast cancer survivors who race dragon boats report growth in greater numbers than the one-half to two-thirds of trauma survivors who generally report growth.

In 2011 McDonough published another small study, in which she delved further into the experience of dragon boat racing and particularly the social relationships and support that it helped to foster. Since social support is highly correlated with growth, she thought that the relationships might help to explain the large bump in growth she'd found earlier. Oddly, what she found was that these women were not there for support at all. The women were there for something else: to train, to paddle, and to compete. Breast cancer was always in the background, but it was secondary to the team and the sport. "You are not going on a Thursday night to discuss cancer but are going and doing an athletic activity with other cancer survivors," says McDonough. "Now you have a group that you can talk to, the social support is there, but it is a secondary pathway to social support. A lot of participants appreciate that the focus is on the athletics. It gives them a positive focus on an activity." The support is always there if it's needed, but it's in a context of positive athletic achievement. And because these women have been through the same things, they are quick to help and support each other.

These teams are also filled with women who have been through cancer who are fit and healthy and have a positive attitude. They abound with role models, people to aspire to be like, who have found a path to growth and who can show others that they, too, can grow. They are able to have some control over their bodies again, becoming healthy after such long periods of being and feeling unhealthy and weak. "The women don't say, 'I'm glad I had breast cancer,'" says McDonough. "Instead they say, 'Here is something good that has come from this struggle. I might wish it hadn't happened but something good came from it.'"

Since joining the team, Maloney has gone from paddling to becoming a member of the coaching staff to steering the boat and back to paddling. With each move she has been pushed to learn and change and find new strengths in herself. "One of the things that has definitely emerged in me is that I am a leader. I found it in my professional life and in my personal life alike," she says. "I think other people's perception of me has changed a bit, too," says Maloney. "There is a little bit of respect that I do it, that I commit so much time and work really hard." She has experienced the joy of competing and wining races. The sport continues to open her up to new experiences and ways of understanding her own capabilities and potential. "The idea that we could go to an international competition, I never thought about that stuff before in my life but that is possible now," she says. "There are new goals being put in front of me and new things for me going up the ladder to higher levels of achievement. And that is exciting."

After practice that Saturday morning, Maloney stood on the dock talking with one of the coaches. At the upcoming world championship races in Sarasota, Florida, only competitors would be allowed on the boat. That means that the team members would need to take over the tasks of steering and calling out the strategy to their teammates—when to settle into a rhythm, when to push that pace faster, when to sprint for the finish.

Maloney might be tapped to call out the pace. And if so, she'll need to do it while seated in the middle of the boat and paddling. It's a position of great responsibility—if she gets it wrong it can cost them the race. And it's not easy. She'll need to keep an eye on a watch so she doesn't tell her boat to sprint too early or too late. And figuring out how to look at a watch while gauging the race and paddling all at once is causing her some concern.

She took a few minutes to discuss with her coach where she might put the watch, how she'd keep track of what to do and when to make the calls. Rather than getting stressed out about it, she simply told him, "I'll just have to try it out." And with that she borrowed his watch and started getting ready for the day's second practice.

The Power of the Physical

D. J. Skelton, a young lieutenant just out of the United States Military Academy, was deployed to Iraq in November of 2004. He was stationed near Fallujah on the eve of what would turn out to be one of the bloodiest battles of the war. He had been in the country for only a few weeks when he received a radio report that a patrol had spotted something suspicious. He told them to wait until he and others could reach them. As Skelton and his team neared the patrol, Iraqi soldiers fired. A rocket-propelled grenade hit a concrete pylon holding up a highway overpass. The metal mixed with concrete hailed down on Skelton. At first he felt nothing. Then the pain surged through him. He screamed, but there was little sound. Shrapnel had ripped through his cheek and out through his eye socket, damaging the roof of his mouth, his jaw, and his eye. More shrapnel tore through his chest and stomach. A bullet hit his arm. His leg was injured.

Skelton was evacuated and doctors conducted nearly sixty operations in total. Metal rods replaced bones in his arm and leg. His face was reconstructed. He lost his upper palate and upper jaw. In 2005, the army told him that he would have to end his military career.

But Skelton had no intention of retiring. He had other ideas about his future. Years earlier he read about post-traumatic growth in a journal article. As he was beginning his recovery in Walter Reed, he thought again about what he had read. He reached out to Richard Tedeschi and read more of the research he recommended. Because Skelton understood growth, he realized early on that these terrible injuries might hold something positive for him, that he might find something different, better, as a result. He ignored the army's insistence that he retire and instead he threw himself headlong into his recovery.

After Skelton had improved enough that he was discharged from the hospital, his old civilian friends got in touch and invited him to go rock climbing. Pushing his limits in the wilderness had always been part of Skelton's identity. He started rock climbing when he was six years old. He started BASE jumping in high school. He was excited to get back out in the mountains and reconnect with friends, and to climb. "My friends motivated me to look again at the things that I enjoyed doing through a different lens," says Skelton.

But now climbing was complicated. He had limited use of his left hand. He was unable to sustain an elevated heart rate because of the damage to his upper jaw and palate. He had to learn how to climb one-handed while using that same hand to clip himself into bolts in the rock for safety. "You have to learn what your limitations are, and then what you can accomplish within those limitations . . . and if possible expand those limitations," he says.

At the end of 2006, while Skelton was back at Walter Reed for another surgery, he met a young soldier who had lost both of his legs. This soldier had also been a rock climber before he'd entered the army and was desperate to try the sport again. By the end of the conversation, Skelton had promised to take the young amputee climbing.

"Then I got home and sat on the couch and thought, What did I just do? How does a guy with no legs climb?" He asked everyone he knew, but no one was sure. Then he read about Tim O'Neill, a prolific climber who has logged first ascents and speed records. His brother, Sean, is paralyzed from a spinal cord injury. O'Neill helped him to climb El Capitan in Yosemite National Park, a 3,000-foot-tall granite face, in seven days. Skelton persuaded O'Neill to come back to Washington, D.C., the following week to help them figure out how to help these wounded soldiers to climb.

In the meantime, O'Neill was out ice climbing with a friend in Utah. The friend lost his footing, fell two hundred feet, and died on the ledge where O'Neill was standing. "He exploded on the ledge right in front of me." O'Neill remembers. "I was destroyed. I felt horrible." O'Neill considered canceling his trip but Skelton encouraged him to come. He knew that the wounded soldiers could understand O'Neill's grief and his survivor's guilt—they could help him as much as he could help them. "That weekend showed me the power of coming together to acknowledge weakness, failure, fear, destruction, that type of horror," O'Neill says.

That first weekend they gathered about twenty veterans in a climbing gym. One was blind, another a burn victim. Many had lost limbs. They tried to be safe and to have fun. And, thanks to their willingness to experiment, it worked. One person, who was missing both of his legs, was having trouble using his prosthetic feet on the climbing wall. So they turned his feet around. By using his heels instead of his toes, he was better able to get a stable foothold and push himself up. A blind climber worked with a guide who climbed alongside him. Later that night, over too many beers in Skelton's apartment, Paradox Sports was born.

Today the organization takes wounded soldiers and civilians facing physical and psychological difficulties—everything from traumatic brain injury, PTSD, loss of limbs, and paralysis to blindness and more—to extreme environments, and it teaches them how to climb. It has run trips to climb the 2,500-foot-tall face of Half Dome in Yosemite, Mount Rainier in Washington, and Grand Teton in Wyoming. It runs ice-climbing and white-water rafting trips. Paradox aims for such extreme goals because it wants to cater to those people who really want to push themselves.

"Decisive ownership is key," says O'Neill. "You have decisive ownership when you are in a firefight. You have decisive ownership when you are on the side of a cliff. Many of us choose to hang from the side of a cliff, to navigate treacherous white water, or isolate ourselves in the wilderness, deliberately taking ourselves out of comfort. When you do that, when you decide to struggle, you say, I am going to elect to be challenged. You are enlivened. You have to say there are consequences of making that choice and I am the steward of myself. Owning your life can make choices more immediate and shorten the bridge between who you are and who you need to be."

Though Skelton and O'Neill used their own intuition and personal experience as a guide in creating Paradox Sports, research indicates that physical activity can benefit trauma survivors and can even lead to growth. One review of nearly a dozen studies of combat veterans participating in sports found that athletic programs helped to reduce the symptoms of PTSD, increased well-being, and helped boost active coping, which can help lead to growth. A study of Paralympic athletes found that participation in their sports was linked to post-traumatic growth, particularly when it comes to finding meaning in one's life.

Kate Hefferon, a senior lecturer in applied positive psychology and director of the Posttraumatic Growth Research Unit at the University of East London, studied an exercise class for survivors of breast cancer. In the study, published in 2008, she found that the class was an integral part of what helped these women heal and grow from their experience. The class provided women with a safe environment and a community of others who understood their experience, which allowed them to develop a sense of inner strength and increased self-esteem. Just as important, they developed a healthy lifestyle, which Hefferon says is a change that is not well recognized by the traditional means of measuring growth. The cancer had taught these women to fear their bodies—they were alienated from their own physicality. Regular exercise reconnected them with their bodies and gave them back a sense of control. Whether they knew it or not, Skelton and O'Neill were heading down the right path.

At the start of a Paradox expedition, the group talks about risk management and expectations for the trip. Guides encourage the participants to talk to each other about their experiences. Often an older veteran, a "mentor," helps if issues arise with PTSD. These discussions are not meant to be facilitated group therapy—conversations go where they go. The group eats meals together. There are many staff members to help with the physical challenges that participants face as they scale mountains. And everyone shares their "aha moments," any revelations that people might have had along the way.

That kind of communication, particularly in such an active program, can have real benefits according to Hefferon. Her 2008 study found that the relationships developed in the program were a central element that helped people to grow. Just as in the dragon boat study, these women were able to talk about their problems without feeling pressure to communicate. The reason for their expanding social network was the exercise, but within that context they got to know other cancer survivors who were doing well and had grown, which has been shown to aid in growth. Dragon boat racer Maloney benefited from just that kind of dynamic with her team and Paradox Sports creates a similar dynamic among its participants.

"Meaning is crucial to what we do," says O'Neill. "We are big promoters of people looking for meaning in life." And the meaning that people find in the wilderness, the lessons they learn, quickly translate back to their lives at home. "You have to be present in the situation on a climb. You need to make the right decisions to promote well-being. It should be a short bridge to take that lesson back to home. People turn around and want to be mentors to give back," says O'Neill. "People often say that they did not know until they had this experience that they had this power."

It's Not the Destination, It's the Journey

In the fall of 2013, Kurt Volker arrived in Grand Teton National Park for a Paradox Sports trip. Volker, an air force mechanic who worked on F-15 fighter jets and joined the military in 1991, struggled with a range of disabilities from his two decades in the service. He suffered terrible pain from a back injury as well as dizziness and memory loss. Nonetheless he was excited at the prospect of scaling the 13,766-foot peak, or at least trying to.

That first morning in Wyoming, Volker met five other veterans who were planning to climb with Paradox. They talked and got to know one another. He was happy that he found others who were struggling, others who were hoping to reconnect with their youthful adventures in the wild just like he was. But things did not start out well. Before the climb the groups would spend two days training. And the second day they would be rock climbing. Volker knew that this would be a challenge.

As Volker started up the first pitch that morning, it quickly became apparent that he was going to have a tough day. The positions Volker needed to get into and the strain he needed to put on his legs to climb began to cause him pain. He was starting to get dizzy. Nonetheless he forced himself to keep going. "I decided I was going to push through and give it all I had. I was tired of failing," he says. He made it up that first pitch, but it was a struggle.

During a short break between the sections of rock, he caught his breath and talked with the guide. He decided he'd try for another. "I was halfway up the second pitch and I got dizzy. I wanted to puke," he says. He wanted to go down, but the guides told him it was easier for him to go up than to go down. While Volker fought his dizziness and tried to decide whether he wanted to continue up or head back down, the guide stepped over him and started up the next pitch. "If he is going up, what choice do I have?" Volker thought. "I can't go down myself. I pushed through. I took it one foothold, one handhold at a time." The guide did the same thing at the bottom of the next pitch. Before Volker knew it he had managed to power himself up five challenging rock faces.

He sat at the top, looking out over a nearby lake. "How did that happen? How am I on top of this thing?" he asked himself. "That was a life-changing moment. Realizing that I can get past my stuff, my whole psyche changed. Everything about me changed."

Volker grew up in New Jersey. He was very active. He ran every day. He was a mountain biker and a backpacker. He loved being in the wilderness and pushing his physical limits. Before joining the air force he was an outdoor educator, leading camping, climbing, and canoeing trips. He joined the air force and became a jet plane mechanic. In 1998, a head injury left him with memory problems but he continued his work.

Shortly after his injury, Volker was sent to Turkey. The United States was bombing northern Iraq in Operation Desert Fox. His skills were in high demand to keep the F-15 fighter jets airborne. Often Volker had to repair or replace components in the four-and-a-half-foot-high space underneath the jet. Rather than use a jack stand to raise the components back into place so they could be bolted back on, he found it much quicker to simply boost the heavy equipment into place with his back and shoulder. A colleague would then bolt it into place. His planes never missed a mission due to mechanical problems. "I worked with forty guys and I did not want to let them down," Volker says. "I wanted to be that role model who did whatever it took to get the job done."

But in the process Volker was destroying his back. He retired from the air force in 2011 and then had surgery to fuse two vertebrae. Then his health problems began to accumulate. Because of his head injury his short-term memory can disappear with little warning. He gets lost in his own bedroom, forgetting which door leads out. He forgets where he's going when he drives. "I have to stop and sit and calm down and it comes back," says Volker. "It only lasts for a short time, but it is long enough to know that you have no control over it."

Volker has been diagnosed with Ménière's disease, which has given him bouts of vertigo and caused him to lose hearing in one ear. He likely damaged nerves in his spine by waiting so long to have his bulging disk operated on and was in terrible pain following his surgery. "When you have a disability, you lose your identity. I can't run.

That was a huge outlet for me and it was a big deal to lose it. I walk slower than an old man," he says. "For someone who has dedicated everything to being so active, to not be able to be in it anymore is a crushing blow. It changes everything about your life, your relationship with your wife, your kids. You are pissed-off at the world."

Then Volker heard about Paradox Sports. The organization's trips really appealed to him. It was a way to reconnect with the activities he loved before joining the air force, to find a way to be active again. "I was really hemming and hawing," says Volker. "I didn't want to go there and find out that this is something else I can't do. I was already up against so many things that I couldn't do, finding another one would be a big blow. I didn't want to get pushed down into a funk, a depression." Finally he made the call to Paradox Sports and set out for Wyoming.

When Volker awoke in his cabin on the morning the group planned to ascend the mountain, he felt terrible. His leg and back hurt. He was still getting dizzy spells. "I felt like I'd been run over by a steamroller," he says. That day the group planned to hike to a hut over 11,000 feet up the mountain and then make the final push to the summit the following day. Because of the altitude, Volker would not be able to take his pain or vertigo medication. He desperately wanted to make it to the summit. But he also did not want to put anyone at risk if he couldn't make the climb. He knew there was little chance that he would make it to the top feeling the way he did. "I didn't want the whole team to suffer because of me," he says. He went with the group to the trailhead, listened to the briefing, and then watched as the group walked up the path without him.

As he hiked down off the mountain, he ran into Paradox Sports cofounder Tim O'Neill coming the other way to join the rest of the group for the push to the summit. O'Neill had heard about Volker's remarkable effort the day before. The two had never met, but O'Neill gave Volker a huge, long hug. He told Volker not to worry about the summit. Climbing, he said, is all about the journey. And though it was an old cliché—it's not about the destination, it's about the journey—something about that hit home for Volker.

Volker returned home. He was miserable. He'd never failed at anything he set his mind to before. Here was one more confirmation of what he had lost, what he would never be able to attain again. But at the same time, somewhere in the back of his mind, that idea that O'Neill planted—it's about the journey—stuck with him. When winter rolled around and Paradox opened up spots for its trips later that year, Volker signed up for the Teton trip again. "My wife was one hundred percent against it. She saw the devastation in my face when I came back home last time and there was no way she wanted us to go through that again if I went and didn't make the summit again," says Volker. But he had begun to think differently about this new trip and about his failed attempt last time. If he signed up again, he thought, that would change the way he thought about the previous trip and his failure to climb to the summit. If he tried again, that first trip wouldn't necessarily be a failure. Instead it would be training, part of the process, part of the journey required to make it to the summit.

Over those months since his failed attempt to climb Grand Teton, he had been thinking a lot about his life—deliberately ruminating. He thought back on his career in the air force, the deterioration of his body, the lapses in his memory, and the frustration he had with all his physical failings. He realized that he had to let it all go. "You have to get on that journey to find the new you. If you don't find the new you, you are going to die. You have to find the new you, that is the journey," says Volker. "It is amazing. It saved me."

Volker went back to Grand Teton in 2014. He didn't make the

summit this time, either, but he made the first stage of the climb to the hut on the mountain at over 11,000 feet. This time he was not disappointed. Instead he was amazed. "I've never climbed that high before in my life when I was able-bodied, but now I have chronic pain, vertigo, and now I get to eleven thousand feet?" he says. "If I made it that far last year, I can make it to the summit this year. It is about the journey, meeting cool climbers, hanging out, meeting more vets. Maybe I'll meet that guy I was three years ago."

Volker is planning more climbing trips this year, perhaps to Idaho or even overseas, the Andes or maybe the Himalayas. He is amazed at how lucky he is to even be considering these trips. He also volunteers with the Wyakin Warrior Foundation, an organization that provides mentoring, professional development, funding, and other services to veterans. The veterans he mentors can call him for advice twenty-four hours a day. He understands how they grapple with the loss of their identities—their identities as soldiers and as strong, able-bodied, athletic people. Volker says that now he is in a position to help them find a new sense of self, in just the same way that Skelton and O'Neill helped him.

"It feels really good to help," he says. "I lost a part of me when I got out of the military and it took a bunch of people to help me to get to where I am now and fill that void. It was life changing, truly. I talk about Paradox Sports every day. They saved me from myself, saved me for my family."

CHAPTER 11

Bonding with Those Who Get It

How the Sad Dads Saved Each Other

WHEN SCOTT KENNEDY WAS IN HIS EARLY THIRTIES, HE FELT LIKE he was on top of the world. He lived in New York City. His job at the drug company Pfizer paid well. He fell in love and got married. Soon he and his wife had a baby, a son named Hazen. "I felt like I had arrived. I knew what I really wanted in life," says Kennedy. "I felt like this was the pinnacle."

The first few years of Hazen's life were fun, blissful, harried, what every first-time parent of a young child goes through. Hazen started preschool when he was three years old and seemed to love it. He was talkative, energetic, and social. Then, one day, Kennedy got a call at work from Hazen's teacher. Hazen was acting strangely. He was sitting by himself, not talking at all. He was lethargic and had been constipated. Kennedy picked up his son from school and took him to the pediatrician. By the next day his son had not improved so the couple took Hazen to the hospital. The doctor noticed that Hazen's stomach was distended, which prompted him to order an ultrasound and to run new tests. Kennedy was waiting to get back to work when the doctor returned and pulled a curtain around them for privacy. He told Kennedy and his wife what he'd found: Hazen had cancer. "My whole world fell apart," says Kennedy.

Hazen was diagnosed with neuroblastoma, a rare pediatric cancer—only about 650 cases appear in the United States each year. Neuroblastoma can be hard to diagnose and, because it often spreads quickly, it is hard to treat. Children undergo powerful chemotherapy treatments. Bones can become brittle, and children are often in horrible pain. Mortality rates are very high—only one in three survive. Hazen had emergency surgery that day. The surgeon was unable to remove all of the cancer so, just four days after his surgery, while Hazen was still unconscious and recovering from surgery, doctors began chemotherapy. But the chemotherapy was not completely successful, either. Cancer remained in Hazen's liver, in his bone marrow, and elsewhere in his body.

The surgery had been very invasive and the chemo had weakened the three-year-old. Hazen had to go to occupational therapy to relearn how to use his hands and work on basic motor skills that had been compromised by the surgery and the months in bed. He had to go back to using a diaper and had to eat through a feeding tube. Kennedy and his wife rarely left their son's side those first months. Friends brought them food and sat with the young boy so Kennedy and his wife could sleep. "We had a really amazing support group," says Kennedy.

Finally, three months after his surgery, Hazen was released from the hospital. When the family arrived back at their apartment building in the Hell's Kitchen neighborhood of Manhattan, fifty people were waiting outside with signs welcoming Hazen home. But being at home presented new challenges. Hazen still needed to eat through a feeding tube. Kennedy and his wife had to check the machine to make sure that it was working properly, make sure the port was sterile, and feed him using the tube. Hazen continued to use diapers. Every night they went through two hours of medical procedures. And they were in and out of the hospital on a regular basis. Through it all they had to maintain a positive attitude around their sick son.

"You have the regular physical caring and the emotional caring; it is so tuned up and so intense that you get so close. We believed that we were closer to our kid than normal parents," says Kennedy. "We are able to share the highest highs." Kennedy remembers every detail of the first day that he and Hazen went to Central Park after he was released from the hospital. "It was such a simple thing, we went and got an ice cream. It was incredibly joyful. We were crying and hugging," says Kennedy.

Those moments were particularly powerful because Kennedy and his wife didn't know when they might end. Every night Kennedy, who is not religious, would go outside his apartment building and stand on the sidewalk looking for a star. In Manhattan, a dense, glowing city where the nighttime sky never really looks dark, it could take him ten or even fifteen minutes to find one. When he did, he said the same prayer on that star each night: "I am not asking for much, just for him to get through this night."

Kennedy and his wife tried to talk about the illness with Hazen in a way that he could understand while avoiding loaded words like *cancer*. He knew that he had bad cells in his body and that they were trying to get those bad cells to go away. When people asked him why he had no hair or no eyelashes or asked about his feeding tube, Hazen was always direct. He was trying to get rid of the bad cells, he'd say, and the medicine was making him lose his hair. "He'd charm them and say, 'Isn't my head shiny,'" says Kennedy. "The smiles he had were the biggest smiles I've ever seen."

It soon became clear that the treatments were not working. The remaining cancer was not going away. The Kennedys researched new, promising treatments, looking for anything and everything that might push the cancer into remission. They quickly discovered a listserv, or email group, of parents of children who'd been diagnosed with neuroblastoma. They shared tips on new drugs, trials, different treatments they could talk about with their son's doctors or try to pursue. They found a supportive group of parents, many of whom were going through the same emotional disaster as Kennedy and his wife. They clung to the time they had with Hazen but were terrified because his condition wasn't improving. "As a parent, your whole purpose is to protect your child. When you see your child being tortured over a multiple-year time frame, it is . . . I can't describe it," says Kennedy. "There is nothing worse that a human can go through."

One Friday, in November 2007, Kennedy walked his son across Central Park to the hospital for his routine outpatient treatment. But the visit turned out to be anything but routine. Hazen's liver was failing. He had sepsis, a potentially lethal reaction to an infection, and other complications. There was nothing more the doctors could do. "Everything came crashing down. Everything," says Kennedy.

If there was nothing else to be done, Kennedy knew that they would all rather be at home than in a hospital room, so they went back to their apartment. For three days Kennedy ran back and forth to the hospital in a desperate effort to find any effective treatment for Hazen, but nothing helped.

Hazen died at home on the daybed in their living room just as the sun was setting. Afterward Kennedy sat in a chair next to that daybed for what must have been twenty-four hours. "I stayed in that chair thinking, I don't want any time to pass. I want to be frozen now in the moment. I am so full of him, of my son. I thought, I am five hours away from him being alive with me. I don't want to be farther away than I am right now. I couldn't get up. In my mind I could stay there forever and never leave," says Kennedy. "In an instant, you are not a parent anymore. It's an unbelievable thing to wrap your head around. You are a parent and then you are not a parent."

The Power of Virtual Support

Kennedy had become close with a number of the parents on the neuroblastoma listserv. Eight people he knew through the listserv from all over the country came to Hazen's funeral. "Those are the people that my wife and I spent time with at the service, not other people that came," says Kennedy. "They were our community, our lifeblood."

Kennedy had few other people that he wanted to turn to. His mother was suffering from Alzheimer's disease when Hazen died and she was not able to provide any support. Interactions with friends became awkward and Kennedy often became bitter and angry. "They don't know what to say because losing a child is hard. You can't do the normal greeting card sympathy statements," says Kennedy. Friends would often tell Kennedy and his wife that they would eventually get over it. "As soon as I heard that I would go out of my mind," Kennedy says. "I don't want to get over it. It's not possible." About a week and a half after Hazen died a group of friends pushed Kennedy to go out to dinner with them just to get him out of the house. During dinner one of his friends said something that Kennedy thought was insensitive—he doesn't even remember what—and he stormed out of the SoHo restaurant onto the sidewalk. He screamed as loud as he could. And then he kicked a garbage can. He kicked it so hard that he broke his foot. "So that is where I was when I first went out in public," he says with a bit of a laugh.

Kennedy and his wife tried going to a support group for grieving parents. An hour into it they fled the room feeling like there was no way they could talk about their feelings with a group of strangers. Eventually Kennedy went to a therapist. He found someone who would just let him open up and expose the depths of his grief. His wife went a few times but then stopped, he says. Kennedy talked, not only about his grief, but about his guilt. He thought that he could have caught the symptoms earlier (though even his doctor missed them). He felt that his lack of a sixth sense about his child's health cost Hazen his life. It was horribly unfair that he, a man in his forties, should still be here, alive, when his son, who had his whole life ahead of him, was dead.

The typically upbeat and outgoing man that Kennedy's friends had known for decades disappeared completely. Kennedy became withdrawn and angry. He drank. He was hard to be around. He and his wife stayed together for six months, coexisting in the most basic way, and then they separated. The breakup just heaped more misery on him. "I couldn't imagine life without her; it was like the end of the world," says Kennedy. "She was even more than a life partner; she was the one that I shared this whole experience with and now she is gone. No matter how bad it was, she was my lifeline; she can't go away. I lost my entire family."

Throughout this time, Kennedy kept posting on the listserv. People would check in on him and send supportive messages. He started emailing some of the parents, particularly the fathers with sick children and those who had already lost their children, and soon the fathers started a separate group. They became incredibly important to Kennedy. Though he hadn't met most of these people in person, they, more than anyone else, understood him and what he was going through.

Kennedy is lucky that he found them. Evidence shows that participating in these kinds of online communities helps trauma survivors of all kinds. A 2008 review of studies of those using online support groups found that participants benefited from an improved sense of well-being, self-confidence, and control and that participation could lead to a sense of increased empowerment. Another study of those with breast cancer and other ailments found that those who used online support groups showed increased optimism, control, and self-esteem.

A 2012 study of Iraq and Afghanistan War veterans found that combining online cognitive behavioral therapy with communication through an online peer-to-peer support group helped lower levels of depression and helped curb symptoms of PTSD. The University of California, San Francisco's Shira Maguen says that many of the soldiers that she works with have found great benefits from participating in online forums. "These online communities are a way of getting the benefits of a group therapy session, talking vet to vet," she says. "Because they have the anonymity, they don't have to worry about what friends or family may think. They can talk honestly without the fear of judgment."

Because the other fathers in this new online group had sick children or had already lost them, Kennedy felt that they could understand him. And he felt free to express himself however he needed to. There was no filter or inhibition and he was never judged. With this group he could simply be himself and get the support that he needed. Though this group started online, it was about to become far more than a virtual means of support for all of the dads involved, thanks to a chef who delivered dinner to another grieving father.

Finding a Like-Minded Community

One of the other dads on the listserv, John London, knew all too well what Kennedy was going through. His daughter, Penelope, was diagnosed with neuroblastoma when she was just sixteen months old. She lived with the disease for years, sometimes in horrible pain. "When she was sick the pain was so acute, it felt like I was being stabbed in the stomach," London says.

London was one of the fathers who broke off with Kennedy to form their own online group. As London's daughter's condition deteriorated, he called another father in the group, Sydney Birrell, almost daily. Birrell came to New York from his home in Canada to visit the hedge fund manager and his daughter every month and helped however he could.

Several years earlier, Birrell's son, James, had been diagnosed with neuroblastoma. James had six months of intensive chemotherapy. He had a bone marrow transplant. The treatments appeared to work. He went into remission. Everyone was hopeful they'd beaten the disease. Then, seventeen months later, the cancer returned. Doctors can't do much for recurring neuroblastoma. Treatments are largely ineffective. The second round of the cancer was even worse than the first. Growths popped up everywhere, even pushing up beneath the skin on his head, sometimes growing a centimeter in a day.

Just like Kennedy, Birrell went through devastating lows and soaring highs with his son. James had long wanted to compete in a soapbox derby. Birrell entered him in one and James made the finals. James talked on the phone with his favorite actor, Tom Hanks, who sent him cards and notes of encouragement. James would, out of nowhere, make wise and funny comments. Once, on a two-hour drive home from the hospital after a long day of miserable tests and treatments, Birrell noticed that his son was in a good mood. "How do you stay this cheerful?" Birrell asked his then seven-year-old son. "Ya can't let cancer ruin your day," he replied, and then made several farting sounds with his armpit. It was the perfect response.

Back before the era of blogs, Birrell wrote emails at night when he couldn't sleep. He sent them out to family and friends. They would often forward them along to others. Eventually his writing about the horror and frustration of the cancer and his wonder at his son's fortitude reached a huge audience. Responses poured in. "I would get email from people that I didn't know, and it would give me a bit of comfort and support as I struggled with the latest catastrophe," says Birrell.

During the last month of his life, James was in so much pain and so sensitive to any pressure at all that his parents couldn't hug him. They couldn't even hold his hand or kiss him as he suffered and died. Birrell hoped that he could use his experience to help London and others who had to stand by while the disease ravaged their children.

London got desperate as his daughter grew weaker. He pursued experimental treatments. One of them extended his daughter's life for a year and eventually it went into clinical trials to help other children. But it and the other treatments couldn't save her life. Two months before her fifth birthday the cancer killed her.

London was destroyed. "My family and friends were trying to be supportive but they had no idea what I was going through. I would have said that no one on earth could have felt worse than me. I was struggling to just stay alive," says London.

A concerned coworker hired a chef to prepare meals and bring them to the family once a week. One night the chef mentioned that he had also delivered dinners for another father who had lost a child to the same disease and that the father lived nearby. London knew that it was Kennedy from the fathers' email group. The two had corresponded while their children were both alive. Hazen had died just six months before Penelope. Hoping to find someone else who could understand his grief, London got in touch with Kennedy and asked him out for a beer.

The pair drank and talked for hours in a dark Greenwich Village bar that night. And as they did, they settled on two things they wanted to do. The first was to start an organization that would allow them to put the knowledge and expertise they had gained advocating for their own children to work for others. It could help other parents find better treatments and fund trials of new drugs, pushing the medical and pharmaceutical establishment to be more aggressive, to do more to save their children. And the second was a trip.

London, Kennedy, Birrell, and the other dads from the email group who had lost their children flew to an island in the Caribbean for a week, where London had rented a large house for the six of them. The men shared pictures and videos of their kids. They cried and yelled and even laughed. Some tried to get in fights. They drank. A lot. They slept in the bunk beds in each other's room. "We went through this extraordinary time together, this wash of emotion," says Birrell. "A lot of us discovered that we were not the only ones going through this. We shared these deep feelings and out of that came this camaraderie." Though Birrell's son died about five years before the trip, being with the dads brought everything back for him. Five years is nothing for a grieving parent. The pain lasts a lifetime, he says.

For the fathers it was crucial that this group was all men. It had been hard for them to open up emotionally. But because each of them had been through such similar and horrific experiences, they were able to be honest with each other, to talk about their deepest feelings. They discovered that they were not alone. They also realized that they were particularly upset because of the role that they felt fathers were supposed to play in their children's lives. "Dads feel like they are supposed to take care of their families, that you fix things when they are broken. We were all trying to find treatments, scrambling, going to the hospital, networking with doctors," says London. "There is more a sense of failure for fathers. I felt like I wanted my daughter to forgive me. I felt like I failed her."

The six grieving fathers talked about the details of their relationships with their wives and remaining children. After their children were diagnosed, their wives uniformly lost interest in sex. At the same time the men talked about having an incredible sex drive. They had fantasies about nurses. "Almost all of our relationships were in bad shape with our spouses. We felt alienated from our own children. It was hard to feel love for them. We were just destroyed, our hearts ripped out of our bodies," says London. They discussed wanting to cut themselves off from their parents and siblings because they were too hard to relate to. They drew pictures of their relatives and tore them up. These other grieving fathers were the only ones with whom they could express all of the turmoil they felt under the surface. "To feel safe and have that reassurance is priceless. If you can't get that out, you feel crazy and set apart from the world," says Kennedy. "It makes you feel withdrawn, which you don't need. You need to be out and part of the world and you can't do that with normal people that are not part of this club."

On the island they would go out together, sometimes spending hours eating and drinking and talking. It was an odd sight. People would often ask them who they were, why they were all together. At first they made up stories. Then finally they told someone the truth— they were fathers who had all lost their children to cancer. London said that they were the Sad Dads. And the name stuck. They even made T-shirts. Half a dozen years later they still get together once a year.

Kennedy may have benefited the most from the Sad Dads. Unlike the others, he had no other children. Hazen's death and his separation from his wife left him completely untethered. "Scott's situation was almost insurmountable. He had every right to close the curtain. I don't know why he didn't commit suicide. What kept him alive?" asks Birrell. The other fathers who had surviving children had little choice but to find some way to move on. "We didn't have a choice to check out," says London. Kennedy needed the relationships developed on the listserv, and later, friendships with London, Birrell, and the other Sad Dads. "The Sad Dads were a big factor in keeping Scott going," says London.

The Sad Dads provided these grieving fathers with the kind of social support they couldn't get anywhere else. Outside of this group, they felt like no one could relate to their experience, but within it, they were surrounded by those who understood. "The Sad Dads let Scott share whatever the hell he wanted," says Birrell. "There is nothing like crying and hugging and doing this with your brothers, your Sad Dad fraternity." Birrell's wife, Pam, says the Sad Dads saved all of them, and provided these fathers with a rare, safe place to open up to their emotions. "To see these guys develop this intuitive, supportive, safe place, it is really extraordinary. They talk about just about everything and it is private, it is safe and confidential. They don't judge, they just support each other," she says. "I think that has helped to change who they are, to have that emotional safety."

Psychologists have long been aware of the value that social support provides for trauma survivors. Those with strong social networks report less PTSD and depression. And social support has been linked to growth. But, as Kennedy's experience indicates, it is not just any kind of social support that helps—he found no value in the efforts of friends and family to help him. Support from those who understand what the survivor is going through, who the individual feels he can be open with, provides the most benefit. Trevor Powell, a consultant psychologist with the Berkshire Healthcare National Health Service Foundation in the United Kingdom, has been working with brain injury survivors for twenty-five years. Brain injuries can lead to memory loss, changes in personality, and the loss of cognitive and physical abilities, making them particularly hard on family members. Often those with brain injuries feel cut off from their former lives and have a hard time opening up, in much the same way that Kennedy and London and the other Sad Dads felt cut off from their traditional centers of support.

Powell conducted a study, published in 2012, of traumatic brain injury survivors eleven and thirteen years after their injuries. He found significant post-traumatic growth in the group but also found that those who had the strongest social support reported the most growth, sometimes 50 percent more than others. The most effective type of social support for this group is other brain injury survivors, says Powell. "I am a great believer in running groups with six or seven people together in a room who have all had brain injury. I think this is the best medicine, to meet people who are on the same road as you," says Powell.

Lawrence Calhoun emphasizes that it is the quality of the support that matters most. "The extent to which a person listens to someone, accepts them, that the immediate social response is supportive and accepting of the idea of growth and doesn't slap it down, that is important," says Calhoun.

Healing by Helping Others

When Kennedy went back to his job, his heart and mind were not in it. Instead he kept thinking about the conversation he had with London, about how the two of them might be able to put the knowledge and expertise they gained helping their own kids through the maze of cancer treatments and drug trials to work for other parents. The more he learned about how cancer was treated, the angrier he got. He discovered that there was almost no difference between the survival rate for those with neuroblastoma in 1990 and the day that Hazen was diagnosed in 2005. And, he says, throughout the medical establishment, the bar for success with cancer treatments is incredibly low. If a drug reduces a tumor by 30 to 50 percent, it is considered a huge success. "This is a blockbuster?" he asks. Kennedy says that shrinking a tumor by that much only extends the patient's life and sometimes not by much. The cancer will still kill him.

Instead of doing his job, he spent his time outlining the goals and mission of the organization he wanted to run and talking with London and the other dads about what the organization should do. He never would have considered such an endeavor before Hazen was diagnosed. Like most people he was concerned with the well-being of his family and his own financial stability. "In no way was I giving back," he says. Hazen's cancer and death, Kennedy's grief and suffering, the support that he found from the other Sad Dads changed everything. "I am on red alert all the time," says Kennedy. "That red alert is still on in me and I am going to continue to keep using it for good. I may be a broken man, but a broken man can help somehow." With financial backing from London, he quit his job and the pair founded the nonprofit group Solving Kids' Cancer.

The organization is inside a sixteen-story prewar building in midtown Manhattan that is filled with nonprofits that receive subsidized rent. Kennedy's office is spare—a meeting table, a desk with a laptop computer, piles of boxes filled with files, and a whiteboard. And then there are the pictures: lots and lots of pictures of Hazen smiling, his head bald and shiny. Kennedy shows them off like any proud father would. Seven years after Hazen's death, Kennedy is in a new commit-ted relationship and he and his partner have a four-year-old daughter. He struggles at times to balance his old life, his grief and loss and love for Hazen, with his new family. Being focused on the present sometimes feels like a betrayal of his son, so he tries to talk openly about Hazen and his feelings with his new family. "There are some challenges, but we manage to get by," he says.

His organization—he runs the day-to-day operations and Lon-don is the chairman of the board—works with doctors and research-ers to identify promising and aggressive new cancer treatments for pediatric cancers with high mortality rates. It funds trials. It pushes the medical establishment to demand better outcomes. He is not interested in drugs that simply reduce tumors by 50 percent and he's hoping that Solving Kids' Cancer can help to raise the bar, push-ing the industry to reassess how it defines a successful cancer drug. "We're looking for one hundred percent reduction or survival indi-cators that show that people would go into complete remission," he says. "We invest in those things. What's the point other than that?" He works with like-minded doctors and researchers to identify and fund promising new treatments that have not been tried on children before. At times he has even helped people to bring in risky new treatments from overseas and pushed to get those drugs into trials here. He also helps match families with trials, opening the doors to treatments that they and their doctors may not know about. The or-ganization is responsible for seventeen new treatments for childhood cancer.

This is work that Kennedy never could have imagined doing be-fore Hazen's death. But now, he says, there is nothing he wouldn't do to try to save another child from dying from cancer, to stop another parent from having to endure what he has endured. "Parents like myself have superhuman qualities that you bring out in yourself while caring for a child with cancer," Kennedy says. "I want to use these qualities to help save lives. No one turning a negative into a positive does it in a half-assed way."

Kennedy isn't the only Sad Dad to have found a way to turn his child's death into something meaningful for others. After James's death, Birrell's emails were published in a book called *Ya Can't Let Cancer Ruin Your Day*, which has a foreword by Tom Hanks and has become a Canadian bestseller. He and his wife started the James Fund, a nonprofit that helps fund research into cures for neuroblastoma. Birrell and his wife have raised more than $5 million so far. He is a choir conductor and feels that his music can help others, providing an uplifting respite from their suffering. He has also recently been certified to run grief support groups, helping others who have lost children, and he continues to help support parents whose children have been diagnosed with the disease. He still misses his son every day and he doesn't sleep much at all. The grief will never leave, but, he says, "I am a new person. For my wife and I, we try to make the world a better place. It gives us meaning and focus."

Five years ago Kennedy was diagnosed with prostate cancer and had his prostate removed. He now has annual checkups to see if the cancer has recurred but otherwise his own cancer has had little impact on him. He has already experienced so much more in life than his son that his own mortality doesn't strike the same fear in him that it would in most others. He isn't afraid to tell people what he thinks and embraces the people that mean the most to him.

London is amazed that Kennedy has the fortitude to deal with childhood cancer every day. It would overwhelm him, London says, bringing back too much of the grief, the loss, and the memory of his daughter. But Kennedy says that he needs to be immersed in it. He couldn't survive any other way. "I'm exposing myself to huge minefields, trauma, and horror, but this trumps it," Kennedy says. "The ability to save even one life, it makes me navigate the pain and endure it because that one life is the only thing I am reaching for. It's my whole meaning."

CHAPTER 12

Managing Distress and Learning to Grow

The Path to Change Through Therapy

On a January afternoon in 2010, Joslin, a Haitian teenager, was at home with her aunt, her twelve-year-old brother, and a house-keeper who had worked for the family for many years. That was not unusual. Her mother, a nurse, worked long hours and her father, who she says was physically and emotionally abusive, was distant. Joslin (who asked to be identified only by her middle name) had helped to care for her younger brother—the two were very close.

At 4:53 that afternoon a massive 7.0 earthquake hit Haiti. Joslin's family lived on the first floor of a four-story building. The structure was no match for the suddenly lurching ground on which it stood. The entire building collapsed on top of them. Joslin's aunt was decapitated and died instantly. Her younger brother was trapped without enough air and suffocated about fifteen minutes later.

Joslin and the housekeeper were trapped side by side beneath the rubble. Somehow there was enough air for them to breathe, but Joslin couldn't move. Her legs were buried in sand up to her thighs and she couldn't get them out. A door had fallen above her and there were big blocks of concrete to her left. Even if she could free her legs, there was nowhere to go, no way to move. Other injured people were trapped on the floors above her. She heard them screaming. Some screamed for a day. Some screamed for two. And then they stopped.

After days buried beneath the debris, Joslin grew certain that she was going to die. Hope of ever being discovered was fading. There was nothing to do but cry and scream for help. And that is what they did, day after day. Six days after the quake, someone walking by the collapsed building heard them. He went for help. Soon rescue workers were digging through the rubble. Finally, they found Joslin and the housekeeper and pulled them from the building. Miraculously, they had both survived.

The pair were rushed to a temporary hospital run by the University of Miami Medishare program, which was set up to help victims of the earthquake. There she found an uncle, who quickly got in touch with her surviving family members. They rushed to the hospital to see her. "My grandmother, when she heard my voice for the first time after I got found, she passed out," says Joslin. "My whole family was celebrating because for six days, they were just in grief. They couldn't eat, sleep, or do anything. Then they just heard my voice and they just went crazy."

Remarkably, Joslin had few injuries, but the ones she had were terribly infected. The cuts on her left foot were so bad that her foot had to be amputated. Her right leg was also infected but doctors were less concerned about it. And for Joslin, the infection seemed to be a minor irritant, the least of her worries after losing her brother and her aunt, the horror she survived beneath the building, and having her own foot amputated. Aftershocks from the earthquake continued for two weeks—more than fifty of them were over 4.2 in magnitude. "I could feel the ground shake and every time it did all of the images would flash in front of my face. I would start screaming in the middle of the night and wake everyone up," says Joslin. Each time doctors and nurses would rush to her, give her a sedative, and try to calm her down.

Soon the doctors realized that the infection in her leg wasn't clearing up; in fact it was festering and becoming a serious threat. They were forced to amputate her right leg, too. But that didn't stop the spread of the infection. She was getting worse and their best efforts were not effective. In March they sent Joslin and her mother to New York for treatment. Her mother refused to leave her side. "If it wasn't for my mom, I wouldn't be here today," she says.

Though Joslin's body healed in New York, she was overwhelmed by what she had experienced. She had night terrors about being trapped beneath the rubble, about the dead bodies around her. "It's really terrifying," she says. "You are just paralyzed there between a state of being awake but not really awake. You don't really know what's happening. There's like this thing in your chest." Her PTSD was debilitating. Going outside in New York City was unbearable. Tall buildings were everywhere. She was convinced that any one of them might fall on her at any moment. When she heard a song that reminded her of her younger brother, her grief was overwhelming.

At the same time she was struggling with losing her leg and foot and trying to understand who she might be as a disabled person. "I just thought I would be in the wheelchair forever," she says. "I didn't even know that there was such a thing as prosthetics." But with a little prodding from those at the hospital, she gave them a try. The first time she put them on, it changed everything. "There was hope for me to walk again," she says. "There was an adrenaline rush and I was just walking all over. For the first time, I was really, really happy." Within a month of first trying the prosthetics, she was walking with a single crutch, pushing herself to keep trying through the pain.

Joslin moved from the hospital to the Ronald McDonald House, which provides housing for children undergoing medical treatment for serious illnesses and injuries when they and their families are away from home. Finally she found people closer to her own age she could relate to. "These kids, they were really mature because they were suffering on a daily basis. I could understand their suffering, even though mine was temporary, but still we would connect," she says. But soon she discovered the horrible downside to those friendships. Many of the children at the Ronald McDonald House have terminal illnesses. Some of them did not survive for long after Joslin met them. "Some days, I would just question myself. Why was I always surrounded by death? The people that I love the most, they always die," she says. "I thought I was cursed."

Managing Post-Traumatic Stress with Therapy

For a trauma survivor like Joslin, fear, anxiety, and grief can be debilitating. Learning to manage it, to gain some level of control is vitally important. And it is no simple feat. In fact, the response to traumatic events is often so overwhelming that most people simply try to avoid it altogether. Some people try to block memories of the trauma entirely. Unfortunately, that doesn't work. The memories remain and can be triggered with little warning by seemingly unrelated sights, sounds, or smells. Other people protect themselves from the trauma by separating all emotions from the events. But this often leads to behavior problems—the person can act out on those unexamined feelings by hurting themselves or others. And some people simply try to duck the issue entirely, using what is called avoidance—making great efforts to avoid any events or situations that might bring traumatic memories flooding back.

All of these means of attempting to hide from the trauma can help people to handle the initial, overwhelming impact of the event, particularly in its immediate aftermath, when survivors are too fragile to examine and process what has occurred. So people adopt these coping techniques, often instinctively. But none of these approaches are effective long-term strategies for coping with trauma. If trauma survivors hold on to these strategies for too long, their healing process will be thwarted, which can lead to a host of problems.

When Richard Tedeschi and Lawrence Calhoun begin their clinical work with trauma survivors, they use cognitive behavioral therapy—the most common approach to treating PTSD. It is designed to help clients confront the traumatic experience so that they will be less overwhelmed by the event. At the same time it provides the survivors with tools to manage their fear reactions and understand the cues in the environment that may trigger them. While there are many different forms of cognitive behavioral therapy, therapists using it generally ask their clients to confront the trauma in any number of ways, whether through talking or writing or imagining the traumatic event. By going over the events again and again, they eventually become less threatening. In the process, people are also taught techniques for curbing the fear and anxiety these images conjure, so they can control their response. Tedeschi teaches his clients a range of techniques to help them gain control over their symptoms, including breathing exercises—taking deep, slow breaths and holding them briefly—when they feel they are getting overwhelmed by grief or anxiety. Another technique, called sensory prompting, teaches them to focus on their surroundings, noticing what they hear, see, smell, and feel to halt their traumatic memories and to bring them back to their present, nonthreatening environment.

Many trauma survivors also suffer from what's called survivor's guilt. Soldiers, for example, often feel responsible for another's death on the battlefield. They relive the event over and over, dwelling on what they did wrong, torturing themselves by imagining how they could have acted differently to save their friend. And they punish themselves for failing. Tedeschi uses the facts of an event to help the person better understand what has occurred. In this case the therapist might prompt the client to talk through the traumatic event in detail, letting them point out where they think they failed. Together they might review the physiology of trauma. This can help clients better understand their fight-or-flight response, helping them to realize that some responses are hardwired and out of their control. Once the client understands this, he or she can begin to comprehend more clearly what may have been their fault and what was out of their control. When appropriate, survivors can let go of the guilt—they cannot be responsible for something they do not control.

By using these techniques clients can begin taking control of their post-trauma symptoms themselves, something that gives them a renewed sense of control and mastery—a first step toward believing in their own inner strength.

That was the case for Joslin. She and her mother were referred to the Bellevue/NYU Program for Survivors of Torture, a ten-year-old program that provides mental health and other services to the survivors of torture and other traumas. Joslin's psychiatrist, Dr. Asher Aladjem, prescribed her medication to help her sleep and to help her with anxiety. She and her mother worked with a psychologist together and separately.

Joslin also went through the program's twelve-week cognitive behavioral therapy course, which helped her begin to confront her trauma. She learned some skills—breathing exercises and visualization techniques—to help her avoid sinking into panic and despair whenever images of the quake and her ordeal beneath the building came flooding back. Joslin found triggers all around her. The subway was the worst. The dark subterranean space, the rumble of the approaching train, brought her right back to the earthquake, to being trapped beneath the building. But with breathing exercises and visualization she was able to regain control and eventually she became used to riding the train.

That was a huge step forward for Joslin. And, according to one study by researchers at the University of Miami, that step alone—gaining some control over those feelings of anxiety and despair—can start people on the path to positive change. Researchers studied the impact of cognitive behavioral stress management techniques on a group of one hundred women who had been diagnosed with stage 0 to 2 breast cancer (90 percent of them were stage 1 or stage 2) over the course of ten months. About half of the participants were involved in weekly group therapy sessions that taught them stress and anxiety management techniques, encouraged emotional expression, and helped with social support. The control group was just given basic information about these techniques and a brief introductory meeting.

They found that those who received therapy showed decreased levels of distress, fewer intrusive thoughts about the cancer, and less avoidance of it than the control group. This was to be expected, since these techniques are well-established means of treating those going through such a crisis. What was surprising is that using these techniques showed consistent increases in positive changes as well. Those in the intervention group saw a boost in benefit finding, a broad measure of positive change, compared to their baseline score and compared to the control group. And those results remained elevated each of the three times they were surveyed. It seems that just giving people some tools to manage their anxiety, depression, and other post-trauma symptoms helps them to begin to see some positive changes in their lives.

These techniques are vital for trauma survivors, providing them with some tools to handle their post-trauma responses and helping them to begin to live a more normal and functional life. They may even set people on a more positive path. But Tedeschi is interested in going further, in helping people to achieve growth. "If all people think they can do is try to figure out how to sleep at night or how to go back to work or not scream at their spouse, well, that is all important," Tedeschi says. "But if they think that is all that this is about, there is a big opportunity that is being missed."

Three Therapeutic Paths to Growth

1. The Light Touch

Most of the studies of post-traumatic growth examine people who have changed on their own, without the benefit of therapy or counseling. But clinicians like Tedeschi, Calhoun, the University of Nottingham's Stephen Joseph, and others want to do more than simply let trauma survivors figure things out on their own. They want to help them heal and help them grow. So they have applied what they have learned from their own experiences with clients over decades. And they have been doing a kind of reverse engineering, conducting and reviewing research on how and why people grow on their own to help them determine which therapeutic approaches will help trauma survivors to find new meaning and positive change in their lives.

They have come up with a broad range of techniques. Some are very direct with the therapist outlining clear steps toward growth. Others try to use their expertise to help the person discover their own growth. Joseph is so passive that he sounds more like a Zen master than a psychologist when he discusses his approach.

For Joseph, there is a great difference between the way he approaches a client with post-traumatic stress symptoms and the way many other psychologists might work with that same client. As he sees it, post-traumatic stress is part of the growth process—not a set of symptoms to be cured. That doesn't mean that medication or stress management techniques might not have a place in his treatment. Like Tedeschi, he agrees that patients should be able to discuss their traumatic experience. And he says that patients need to feel that they are in charge of the process. Patients will grow only if they become autonomous enough to find their own means of recovering, reorienting, and moving on to positive change, he says.

Sitting in one of the student cafés at the University of Nottingham Jubilee Campus, which is made up of a collection of colorful and sometimes whimsical modern buildings, Joseph gestures at a group of trees growing on the other side of a pond from where he is sitting. A few are hanging perilously low over the water. One is twisted and rises awkwardly; some look healthy and are growing tall. "Looking at these trees over here, they're all growing," he says. "But some of them don't look in good shape, to be honest. That one over there looks rather sort of spindly and as if it's seen better days, but you wouldn't say it's not growing. And that one's a bit bushier but it's really lopsided. It's practically falling into the water, but it's still growing. So I think there's a way of talking about what growth is, which recognizes that it's not always beautiful and it's not always symmetrical, that it's not always perfect and that it's not always reaching the full potential."

Joseph draws greatly on the humanistic psychologists. He wants to update what Carl Rogers and others were learning about growth in the 1950s and 1960s to address trauma and other more recent concepts. "The growth metaphor for understanding human experience is a model for therapy," says Joseph. Trauma survivors, like all people, are intrinsically growing all of the time, just like trees are growing, he says. Given that, the therapist's role is much like that of a gardener who creates the best possible conditions to enable the tree to grow to its full potential. "We look at that tree over there," he says, gesturing across the pond. "Maybe that's a state of depression. That tree over there, that's obsessive-compulsive disorder, and that tree over there is some sort of post-traumatic stress. There are different ways that these trees are exhibiting distress and dysfunction, whatever it might be. We can come up with ways of describing them, but they're all suffering from the same thing: thwarted growth. And they all need the same thing. They all need what trees need to help them flourish. And it's the same way for people. All people need pretty much the same things to flourish. They need warm, loving companionships, relationships where they're not being controlled, and the space to grow. That is the basis of psychotherapy."

For Joseph, the nature of the relationship between the client and the therapist is very important. "You have to have an unconditional relationship with that person where you are there in a way that supports their agency and autonomy," he says. "Unless you hold that attitude of unconditional acceptance for the other person's journey, it is going to be very hard."

2. Tedeschi's Middle Path

Tedeschi takes a more active role in the process than Joseph. His is a sort of middle path that uses the model he and Calhoun developed to describe the growth process and their research as a guide. Early on Tedeschi and Calhoun identified deliberate rumination—an active thought process that helps one understand one's life, the trauma, and the change that it has wrought—as a central process that allows people to grow. Part of what Tedeschi does in therapy is to help clients begin that process of deliberate rumination and help them think about their personal narratives.

Tedeschi asks his clients to create a timeline of their lives, one that points out the good and bad things that have happened to them, including the traumatic event. This helps his clients begin to work on a narrative approach to their post-trauma recovery—telling the story of who they are and how the trauma changed them. He may prompt them to think about how they have changed throughout their lives. This can help adults, who often have a static view of themselves, understand that they have indeed changed a lot—perhaps they had a rebellious teenage phase or a seeking phase in their twenties, maybe they changed careers or divorced and remarried. It helps prime them for the idea that they may be in store for another life change. And it can help them see that adults do continue to change and grow throughout their lives. This process can also help to start a discussion about how they viewed the world before the trauma. Then, in time, the discussion could naturally move toward how the trauma has upended their understanding of themselves and the world around them. Ultimately the goal is to let the clients decide how their identity, their sense of the world, can be reinvented.

"We try to focus on the aftermath of the event rather than the event itself," says Tedeschi. "The event is a catalyst for a cascade of reactions, and we are interested in what people make of all of that—and how, as a result of that cascade of reactions, there is a real rebuilding opportunity."

Many psychologists say that growth needs to be handled carefully. Push it too soon or too aggressively and clients are easily alienated. Who wants to be told they should be growing when they are in so much pain they can't function? Making clients believe that they should be strong, even when they are in mental agony, can cause them to reject the idea of growth entirely and may even thwart their desire to continue with therapy.

With that in mind, therapists hoping to cultivate growth this way try to provide an environment in which clients can find their own path toward meaning and positive change. That may include helping clients to see the ways in which they are already talking about growth, but never forcing the idea on them. Tedeschi sees the therapist as an "expert companion," someone who can listen to people talk about themselves, their actions, thoughts, and identity before, during, and after an event. In that way the therapist can help their clients see the positive things they may have mentioned along the way. For example, a therapist might help a survivor recognize that he often speaks of his own strength during a traumatic event. If, for example, the person was able to call 911 or flag down help after a traffic accident, that quick action may have helped to save a life. Perhaps the survivor can begin thinking about how he acted and see the inner strength he displayed. That may set the survivor on a path where he recognizes strengths and abilities that he may not have been aware of before.

Much of the approach that Tedeschi and others take is to be a good listener, to try to hear clues in the conversation indicating when clients are noticing changes in themselves and what kinds of changes those might be. Tedeschi lets growth come from the individual, helping the clients identify it on their own. For example, if a client lost a spouse, he might guide the individual toward talking about what he liked best about his spouse. Then, later, Tedeschi might prompt the client to think about what he might do in his own life that would honor the memory of the dead spouse. Tedeschi points out the seeds that are already there, helping the client to recognize the kernels of his own growth.

In fact many therapists who work with trauma survivors say that their clients often bring up positive changes on their own. "They start thinking, I can't feel this crappy forever. What am I going to do with the rest of my life?" says Catherine Whiting, a psychologist at the Seton Medical Center in Austin, Texas, who has worked with cancer patients for most of her career, including Matt Cotcher, the runner who had a brain tumor. If the patient is progressing and is no longer in distress, then she says over time she may push a little if they are not talking about growth on their own. "I might say, 'Death is more in your face than anyone else right now, but you are alive. What do you want to do with your time?'" she says. Often patients are already starting to think that way even if they have not articulated it.

3. A Therapeutic Push

If Stephen Joseph is the Zen master of growth therapy, then Stephanie Nelson is a bit like a drill sergeant, spelling things out simply and directly, leaving no room for misinterpretation or chance.

Nelson first learned about post-traumatic growth when she volunteered in a domestic violence and sexual assault crisis center as an undergraduate. Growth made sense to her. She saw it in the women she met in the center. She thought that traditional approaches to treating trauma were lacking. "People talk about the why factor, why did this happen to me," says Nelson. "Post-traumatic growth helps people to answer those existential questions. It helps people figure out ways they can grow from their experience, which is important to cognitive processing."

After earning a master's degree in social work, Nelson joined the army. In 2011 she was deployed to Iraq as a social worker with the 3rd

Brigade Combat Team, 1st Cavalry Division. She was in an unusual position for someone counseling trauma survivors: she was alongside her clients in the midst of the ongoing trauma. Often she saw clients in between missions, after one trauma and before heading out to the possibility of another. Many of the soldiers she counseled were still coping with traumatic experiences from deployments five or six years earlier. Many had childhood traumas that were exacerbated by their battlefield experiences. She had little time to work with each soldier, so she developed a compressed program that would unfold over five sessions that focused soldiers very quickly on the concept of growth.

Nelson had soldiers make a list of their traumatic experiences to determine which one haunted them the most, prioritizing the most troubling one and then working down the list. Childhood traumas, those involving sexual or physical abuse, were the most complicated and took the most time and effort to address, she says, because of the mix of shame, anger, and guilt. She used exposure-based therapy, asking the clients to recount the trauma over and over until it was no longer so overwhelming and powerful. And she focused the clients toward growth, to help them discover meaning in their experience and channel their emotions into something positive. "I try to give them a more hopeful picture instead of telling them they will have chronic PTSD for the rest of their lives," she says.

One soldier Nelson counseled had to shoot a girl who had a bomb strapped to her. "He could not get over why this child had to die," Nelson says. When he left the service, the soldier started doing volunteer work with children. Later he became a teacher. "It became a way to honor the lives of those who had passed on, to live his life in a meaningful way," Nelson says. "It does not make what happened right, but it is a way to take the energy and channel it in a productive way."

Nelson has since left the army. But she continues to work as a contractor to the military, working with special forces soldiers. Since her time in Iraq she has adapted her program to be used over more sessions. But she still takes a very structured approach, and she is quick to mention the idea of growth early on. Nelson calls her system Growth Path Therapy and growth is discussed in the opening of the book that she wrote detailing the therapeutic process. She makes it clear that clients will struggle, that what they are going through and their effort to heal will be hard. But she also wants them to understand the whole process. She discusses the hero's journey, telling soldiers that they must go through the "dark forest" to get to the other side, that they will find strength and wisdom from facing their fears and confronting their trauma. "I like to give them some hope," says Nelson. "I am asking them to do some difficult work in therapy and I want them to know that there is light at the end of the tunnel, that there is a road map and they are headed towards growth."

Nelson outlines a four-step process: Deal, Feel, Heal, and Seal. In the first phase she urges her clients to confront their traumatic experience using the kinds of cognitive behavioral techniques that have been proven effective and she teaches them stress management techniques. In the Feel stage she helps her clients not only to become comfortable with the memories of their traumatic experience but also to feel the emotions associated with those memories. Like Tedeschi, Nelson helps survivors determine which things may have actually been their fault, and which actions or events were out of their control. She uses a metaphor that soldiers understand: hiking up a mountain with a backpack full of rocks. She tells her clients that with too many rocks in their bags, they will never get to the top of the mountain. They need to unpack their bags, look at the rocks, and see which of them they really need to carry—which are misplaced survivor's guilt that they can discard and which are well-placed remorse that they should keep.

Sometimes the issues are complex. She worked with a low-level soldier who was involved in the torture of detainees during the Iraq War. He told Nelson that officers directed him to torture prisoners in an effort to obtain information and find terrorists and he felt remorseful about it. "It was a systemic issue and this guy was the low man on the totem pole. He can't own all of it. He can't take on guilt for the entire issue," says Nelson. She helped him to see his actions in context and to assign a more realistic amount of blame to himself.

Once clients are progressing through this part of the therapy, she moves on to the healing stage, where she asks them to examine the strengths that they displayed in surviving the trauma and in working through the events in therapy. She emphasizes the value of finding meaning in suffering and the benefits of trying to find something positive in these events. It's not a way of justifying the trauma, but given that these things occurred, it is a way of finding something meaningful in that experience.

In the final step, Seal, she helps them to see that their lives are not defined by the trauma, that it can help to shape them, but that it is one event of many in a lifetime. The goal is to be able to put the trauma in its proper place, to learn from it but not be consumed by it.

For Those Who Survived the Worst

The Bellevue/NYU Program for Survivors of Torture, where Joslin was treated, was founded with the conviction that even those who survive the most horrific experiences can do more than simply adapt to PTSD or become functional but damaged—it's designed to help its participants thrive, no matter what they have experienced in their past.

Dr. Aladjem, who cofounded the program, grew up in Israel in the years after World War II when Holocaust survivors from Europe were flooding there, hoping to begin their lives anew away from the horrors of all they had lost. It's an experience that gave him great insight into how trauma changes people. "We had people from everywhere, from the camps in Germany and Poland. Everybody was in the biggest refugee camp in the world. You experience that and you see the resilience and the growth of people that have lost everything and everybody, including their own self-image as people. There was life after that," he says. That experience, witnessing growth in those who had lost everything, is what drove him into his career and is part of the thinking behind the work that he and his colleagues do at the center. They don't only look to help people heal; they use the tools of psychology and psychiatry to help people to grow.

Clinicians at the center take a wide-lensed approach to treatment. They prescribe medication when it is warranted. Group and individual therapy are both available. The center has staff that help with legal issues and immigration status, food, clothing, shelter, and medical care. The stressors on this group—people from all over the world who have been tortured and those like Joslin who have survived other horrific events—go far beyond debilitating responses to overwhelming trauma. Much like Joseph and indeed Viktor Frankl, the program's clinical director, Hawthorne Smith, who is also an assistant clinical professor at the New York University School of Medicine, says that he does not view his clients as sick, even if they are obviously suffering severe post-traumatic stress symptoms. "The person is not abnormal or crazy, they are going through an abnormal or crazy situation," he says. Finding meaning in their experience is a natural step that many patients are able to take. The point is to help patients to regain some kind of control, to realize that their circumstances were extraordinary, that they are reacting in a normal way, that they are not ill, and that they do have the skills and courage to overcome this adversity.

Clients at the center are asked to complete a twelve-week trauma-focused cognitive behavioral therapy program. There is broad agreement that this approach enables people to begin addressing their trauma rather than being overwhelmed by it. The center's team introduces the idea of growth early on. They plant the seed that new and better things may be possible. "We tell them that nothing is easy but that everything is possible," says Smith. "We don't make any promises but we do say that other people in similar circumstances are able to move forward."

Smith lets the clients' needs determine his approach. Some are able to take more direction, to be ushered through the process in a more directed way. Others are not. Some people, he says, will benefit greatly from one-on-one therapy. They may find it hard or impossible to talk openly with others about what they have been through and asking them to do so could be damaging. There are times when a patient may come to his office and simply sit there, unable to communicate at all, or just sob for five minutes or more. Smith may just listen, offer a tissue, just be there without intruding.

He often finds that group therapy works best. Many people at the center come from cultures where there is a tradition of gathering with friends and family and talking things through. A group mimics that comfortable setting. And these survivors have deep common experiences that they are not likely to find in many others. "To hear from someone who has gone through something similar and has managed to shed light on what has been helpful to him or her, that message is so powerful," Smith says. "Members of the group internalize the fact that they are instrumental in the healing and growth of others. Their experience is not just negative; their ability to overcome is valued and valuable." Perhaps most important, there is laughter. In these groups people find humor in things that many others would find horrifying. Laughter helps them immeasurably.

Joslin benefited from all of this. When she showed up, she was in the midst of overwhelming loss. Her brother was dead and so was her aunt. She had lost a leg and a foot. She had lost her country. She was dropped in New York City, where she didn't speak the language, where she knew no one, understood nothing. She and her doctors weren't even sure if she was going to stay in New York long enough to complete the twelve-week cognitive behavioral therapy course. Yet Joslin was stabilized. She and her mother were inseparable and their support for one another helped pull them both through the trauma. "They shared about how much Joslin's brother meant to her, how he loved his life, and how he would have hoped for them to live their lives, to find that strength to live some of their dreams, to honor their family member by moving forward," says Smith.

Joslin has been freed up to go through the kinds of processes that are at the core of growth—the deliberate rumination, finding a new positive narrative, reorienting her life. When she graduated from high school, she took the time to reflect on everything she had been through. She sat down and remembered her whole life from age five up until that moment. "I just realized that I am a very strong person. I'm a very, very strong person," she says.

Since graduating from high school in 2014 she has decided to go to college to become a nurse, in part because nurses are the people who have the most individual contact with patients. She hopes to work for an organization like the Red Cross, providing medical services after a disaster to help those who are recovering from these horrible events just like her. Given all that she has survived, she knows that she can help others in similar situations.

"I don't want to become one of these inspirational speakers. They just go around and tell people, 'Oh, if I can do it, you can do it, too,'" she says. "I want to be the type of person to actually go to someone who's actually suffering and tell them, 'You know what, you can do this. We can all do this if you really want to survive. There's nothing that can get in your way. You can do it.'"

She has regained her exuberance, her sense of humor, and her fun-loving sensibility. "She has friends as opposed to being isolated. She is more about opportunities instead of limitations," says Smith. "She has made meaning of who she is in the world."

Today Joslin is funny and vibrant. She jokes that people are afraid of her because she has a "mean" face. But that isn't quite right. Her look isn't mean so much as it is a bit reserved or guarded, taking a moment to assess the situation, deciding how she wants to engage. When a smile does come across her face, she lights up completely. She is tall and thin and sits at ease with her prosthetic legs (you would never know that her leg and foot were amputated). And she has a kind of self-awareness and thoughtfulness rare in someone her age.

Someday Joslin wants to return to Haiti. "I just have to go there and go to the place that I was dead—because I was dead—and just make peace with myself and see where my brother died. I'll bring some flowers or whatever and just calm myself and then just move on," she says. "That's the last step, I think."

CHAPTER 13

Fulfillment vs. Happiness

Why Growth Can Last a Lifetime

IN 2003, JAKE HARRIMAN WAS A YOUNG MARINE FIRST LIEUTEN-
ant, just four years out of the United States Naval Academy, when he
was shipped to Iraq to be part of the initial invasion of the country.
As American troops pushed into the countryside, Saddam Hussein's
army retreated to make a stand in Baghdad. Hussein's Fedayeen
special forces stayed behind, but not all of them were there to fight.
Instead many of these elite soldiers went door-to-door in the impov-
erished area, offering food—rice, barley, wheat, or other supplies—to
starving farmers if they would fight the Americans. In the early days
of the war, Harriman and his soldiers were ambushed by these un-
trained and poorly armed farmers. What he saw stunned him.

"It was really horrible stuff," says Harriman. "You see unnatural
things, guys flattened by tanks, carnage, body parts everywhere. I remember the first time I saw this it felt like a movie, you know. Then
you see close up this is a real person, then something happens to you,
you just switch off, in your spirit, your soul."

After one particularly tough fight, Harriman and his men dug holes alongside the main road to Baghdad and climbed in to protect themselves while they waited for supplies. They were hungry, exhausted, and terrified. It was just before sunrise. In the darkness and fog, they could barely make out the figures along the road and some of the men were nodding off in their holes because they had been awake for so long. Harriman got up and went from marine to marine, encouraging them, making them laugh, trying to keep everyone awake and alert. They knew Iraqi soldiers were not far away. Despite his show of fortitude, Harriman was not much better off than his men. His eyes ached. His stomach hurt. "I was hot, exhausted, with a knot in my stomach and a tenseness that wouldn't go away," says Harriman.

As he was checking on his men, he noticed a small white car speeding down the road at them. Harriman thought it was a suicide bomber. He grabbed three of his men and ran into the road but the car didn't slow down. He fired a warning shot and the car screeched to a halt. A man jumped from the car and ran at the group, waving his arms. Harriman thought he was going to blow himself up. Harriman screamed at the man in Arabic, telling him to get on the ground. But he didn't listen. The man was frantic.

Harriman was about to shoot the man when he saw a black military truck speeding toward the car. As it stopped, six Fedayeen soldiers jumped out of the back and opened fire on the car. That's when Harriman realized what had happened. This man was no suicide bomber, nor was he a threat of any kind. He was one of those Iraqi farmers targeted by the Fedayeen. And rather than fight for a bag of rice, he had gathered his family and decided to flee, to seek refuge with the Americans, with Harriman. Harriman's men opened fire on the Fedayeen as the man started sprinting back to his bullet-ridden car. Harriman ran behind him as fast as he could. Two or three of the Fedayeen lay dead as the truck sped away.

When Harriman got to the car and looked in, he saw the man's wife and youngest daughter dead in their seats. The man pulled his oldest daughter from the car and held her while she choked on her own blood.

Harriman just stood there, his gun at his side, and wept with the man for what he had lost. "That is the one time where everything slowed down," Harriman says. "Something inside of me just kind of broke."

Harriman deployed again in 2004, this time leading a special operations unit hunting down high-value terrorist targets. By then many Iraqis wanted the Americans out. People were being recruited to blow themselves up. The country was being terrorized by Al Qaeda in Iraq. "During these missions there was a lot of depravity, desperate poverty, a lot of carnage," he says.

Ever since that day on the road to Baghdad, Harriman began to think differently about what he was doing in Iraq. The people he was fighting, the man who lost his family on the road that day, even some of the terrorists he was catching in nighttime raids were simply poor. Many had no particular ideology. They were coerced into fighting for one side or another because they had few choices in life and none of them were good. "That Iraqi farmer could watch his kids starve to death, or strap on a bomb, or he could make a desperate attempt to escape the Fedayeen," says Harriman. "He made a choice and he lost everything in two seconds."

What happened that day, what he had seen since, bothered Harriman deeply. "My time in combat rocked me to the core, to the point where I questioned the things that I held dear: family, faith, love," he says. But, like all too many people in the service, he never felt that he could talk to anyone about what he saw, how it affected him, and the changes he was starting to experience. "Jake was the consummate leader; he never opened up about it. If anything he put more vigor into doing his job," says Billy Knipper, a marine under Harriman's command who was with him the day the farmer's family was killed. Harriman says that as a leader, he couldn't show any weakness or hesitation or questions about the mission. The lives of his men depended on his ability to be decisive and to project certainty. But underneath his show of strength, he was beginning to question his direction in life. "There are a lot of quiet moments in combat," Harriman says. "There is more downtime than anything else, and you get plenty of time to think about things." And combat had given Harriman a lot to think about.

Harriman grew up in rural West Virginia. His father, a Vietnam veteran, was a school bus driver. His mother looked after Harriman and his three younger siblings and the small family farm. They had a garden for vegetables, a cow for milk and butter, chickens for eggs and meat. They hunted deer, rabbits, and squirrels. Though there was not a lot of disposable income, Harriman had a great childhood. And one thing that Harriman knew from his own upbringing was that poor people are not victims. They are remarkably resilient and resourceful. They often don't need much help to turn their lives around.

Harriman passed up scholarships to top schools, at first to go to the University of West Virginia so he could be with his friends. But after a year he realized that he wanted to serve in the military like his father had and so he transferred to the U.S. Naval Academy, where he had previously been accepted. His religious upbringing taught him to help others. His best friend at the academy, Don Faul, says Harriman often tutored other students who were struggling with classes. He thought that he might do something later in life that would allow him to help others but he hadn't put much thought into what that might be or how to achieve it.

The impulse to help others is hardly rare, yet few people actually do it. And even fewer dedicate their lives and careers to it. For Harriman the horrors of combat made the difference. That experience provided the catalyst that drove him to find a way to remake his life. "Combat is like a filter that allows you to see the world in a much more clear way," he says. "You see the absolute worst humanity can produce and the absolute best that human beings can be."

After two years of thought stemming from that moment on the road to Baghdad, Harriman came to believe that terrorism could not be defeated with weapons alone. It is poverty that opens the door for terrorists in these communities. People who cannot feed themselves, who cannot see a better future for their children, who cannot even make basic choices in life are more susceptible to the coercion of Al Qaeda and other terrorist groups. And poverty, he knew, could not be alleviated at gunpoint. He needed to change his life. "I lived through the flames of combat and I made it through to the other end," he says. "I knew what I wanted in life without a shadow of a doubt and now nothing can rock my vision."

In June 2005, after his second tour, he made one of the toughest choices of his life: he left the U.S. Marines.

Harriman began by applying for jobs with aid organizations but quickly found that they had little interest in hiring a former marine. So he went to business school at Stanford. And once he told his story there, fellow students and professors helped him design a plan for his nonprofit, Nuru International, which is now working in Kenya and Ethiopia. It helps farmers raise their crop yields and incomes, improves education and health care, and cultivates leaders in those communities who can take the model elsewhere and replicate the process across their own countries. In time he hopes to take the program to the world's most chaotic and violent places—Somalia, the Central

African Republic, Afghanistan, and others—with the hope that improving the lives of the poorest people will help deter terrorism and bolster civil society.

Harriman uses the best models from other organizations along with input from the community on what they need to address their own problems. Through boosting agricultural production and improving access to markets and banks, he has helped one region in Kenya approach complete financial self-sufficiency. They must. Nuru staff and financing pull out completely after seven years. His program in Kenya is on track to generate enough revenue on its own to support poverty-fighting programs that are serving more than fifty thousand people. It produces enough surplus income for local leaders to start replicating Nuru's work in other communities. The goal is to help these Kenyan leaders to expand the program themselves, spreading the tools and lessons they learned from Nuru to their neighbors. They in turn will do the same.

At first glance, it's hard to reconcile Harriman with the rising young marine he once was. His dirty-blond hair is shaggy and unruly. He's friendly, seemingly easygoing, and laughs easily. He is committed to his work but not dour or preachy. Several of his former marines say he was the best leader they ever had—willing to listen, to put everyone else's needs before his own, and to lead. Harriman is happy about the choices that he's made, about how he's been able to turn his experience and passion into his life's work.

But many would see those choices as a sacrifice. He takes local transportation and sleeps wherever he is working when in Africa—Nuru has no fleet of the Range Rovers that have become so identified with wasteful development programs in Africa. For many years he slept on couches when he came back to the United States to fund-raise—he rented an apartment here only recently. His friends from business school have been very successful, working in banking or with technology firms. Harriman has no interest in that kind of compensation.

"There is an urgency about him. He is very focused, a different Jake," says Faul. "What has really changed is his clarity and resolve and urgency." His friend John Hancox, who met Harriman at the University of West Virginia, has even noticed the changes in his personal life. "He is less patient with frivolity and things that are less important," Hancox says. "He sees how fragile life is, how brief it can be, that there isn't time to waste."

For Harriman the changes are not a momentary diversion. "Of course the changes are permanent," says Harriman. "These experiences are a part of who I am. They have helped shape me to become the man I am today. Reverting back to the person I was before the trauma doesn't really make much sense. The trauma didn't define me—it refined me in a painful process of growth to become a better person than I ever could have been otherwise."

Transformed for Life

Harriman has certainly grown from his experience. The trauma shook him to his core in exactly the way that Tedeschi and Calhoun describe. What he saw on the road that day, his experiences in combat, forced him to reexamine everything about his life. Though, like far too many soldiers, he never felt that he could talk to anyone about what he was going through, he thought about it. In the long stretches of downtime, he engaged in exactly the kind of deliberate rumination that is central to allowing people to grow. And his traumatic experiences gave him the urgency to act on what he discovered. The trauma of combat was at the core of what transformed Harriman from a marine to the leader of an organization working to end extreme poverty. It's been more than a dozen years since that farmer drove his car toward Harriman that day in Iraq, and if anything his resolve, his dedication to his new direction in life, has only increased. Harriman's growth, his change, has been lasting and there is no indication that this transformation will dissipate.

Harriman is set on his direction, but does growth last so long for everyone? The science of growth is only a few decades old, so there are not many long-term studies that examine how post-traumatic growth changes one's life over decades. Do these positive changes dissipate? After the sting of the loss is less sharp, after the horror fades, do we simply revert to our old selves, to our bad habits? Do trauma survivors change over time, grow stronger in some areas, weaker in others?

A series of studies examining post-traumatic growth in people with traumatic brain injuries may provide some clues. Brain injuries can be completely debilitating and very hard for people to adapt to. They can result in the kinds of challenges that Matt Cotcher and Shane Mullins faced: trouble with movement, balance, speech, memory, sometimes cognitive ability. They may heal in time or not. They are very unpredictable. Carol Rogan, a training manager at Acquired Brain Injury Ireland, began looking into the research on post-traumatic growth and noticed that there were a series of studies that showed growth in those with brain injuries. But each of them was conducted at a different time after the injury occurred. All of these studies measured change using Richard Tedeschi and Lawrence Calhoun's Posttrauamatic Growth Inventory—the scale the two developed to help quantify how much positive change in each of the five areas of growth trauma survivors experienced. All of the studies tallied up the amount of change each person reported in each of the five areas. Higher scores indicate more growth. One looked at growth in those who had been discharged from the hospital an average of 6 months prior to the study, another at 7 months after. One more was conducted on those an average of 32 months after their injury. The mean post-traumatic growth score for the brain injury survivors rose from 33.4 at 6 months to 36.5 at 7 months. Then it jumped to 50.9 at 32 months. She conducted her own study of patients an average of 70 months after discharge. The mean score rose again, this time to 53.8. The more time that passed since the injury, the more positive changes that patients were reporting.

One more study looked at changes even later. Trevor Powell, with the Berkshire Healthcare National Health Service Foundation in Reading, England, decided to conduct a study to learn more about growth in those with brain injuries an average of thirteen years after the initial injury. His findings fit right in with the trend that Rogan noticed. Not only had these people maintained their growth, but it was increasing. The mean post-traumatic growth score he found was 64.6, higher than the scores recorded at earlier intervals. "The further down the track you were, the more post-traumatic growth you reported, the more positive attributions they had about their injury, the more their lives became positive," says Powell. Not only was the growth persisting, but it was increasing.

Another study, which has yet to be published, helps to confirm that growth does not fade. One of the first studies to look at positive change after trauma, and one that helped to influence Tedeschi and Calhoun, was the 1980 study on aviators captured during the Vietnam War conducted by Yale psychiatrist William Sledge. In his study, Sledge found that 61 percent of the former prisoners said they had benefited psychologically from their captivity. They had stronger religious convictions, they enjoyed life more, and they got along better with and appreciated others more. Only 30 percent of control subjects—aviators who had not been captured—reported positive changes.

Now Sledge is working with another researcher on a follow-up study. In 2003 they mailed the soldiers who had been queried in 1976 the same questions asking about life changes. The study has yet to be published, but the early results indicate that little has changed. Not only did the POWs perceive the same kinds of positive benefits from their experience almost forty years later, but they still reported the same significantly higher rates of change than the control group. Growth is not a flash in the pan. Instead it is proving to be a dramatic shift that stays with people and changes their lives for the duration.

Many people have found that their changes last decades. Clementina Chery lost her son Louis Brown in 1993 and remains dedicated to her work. Max Cleland's life took a radical turn in 1968 and he has been coping with trauma and discovering growth ever since. And that has certainly been Harriman's experience. A dozen years after that terrible day on the road to Baghdad, he is unwavering in his direction, spurred on by his experience, dedicated to his vision, and happy to work exceptionally hard, even when he has to do things that are uncomfortable. Though he went to business school, Harriman is no salesman. He's a bit shy around wealthy potential donors and feels awkward about asking for money. Yet he is willing to spend much of his time back in the United States doing just that.

On a cold and windy December evening, Harriman stopped in New York City to meet with a group of potential donors. Inside the dark-wood-paneled parlor room of a brownstone on Manhattan's Upper West Side, Harriman spoke about Nuru to a dozen or so people at the home of Joe Gleberman, an advisory director at Goldman Sachs. Many of them were current and former Goldman executives; others were Stanford Graduate School of Business alumnae. Each of them certainly had the means to help Nuru to continue and to expand its work. And all of them were captivated by Harriman's message.

Gleberman had met Harriman nearly a decade ago, when he was still a student at Stanford. He was intrigued by his ideas and by his story. But Gleberman has met lots of well-meaning people with great ideas looking for money and support. And the vast majority of them do not last long in the nonprofit world. He wanted to see if Harriman would be able to stick with his organization, whether he would have the perseverance to build it up and see it through. Now, all these years later, Gleberman says, there is no doubt that Harriman is set on his direction in life, that he is committed to his work. And Gleberman wants to help.

Wearing a suit—one that a donor took him shopping for—Harriman told his story, about the horrors that he saw on the road to Baghdad that day, about how in an instant that Iraqi farmer lost everything and how in that same instant his own life was set along a different path. "When I go to bed every night, I see the eyes of that farmer on Highway Seven," he says to the group. "And it simply won't go away. It haunts me. And that drives me every day when I get up. We have to push, we have to solve this problem."

Harriman's new life, his focus and determination to help others, also comes with struggle. His tours in Iraq are still with him. He rarely sleeps more than four hours a night. He has trouble opening up to people and that has thwarted many of his romantic relationships. The horrors that he witnessed have not faded with time. But that experience, terrible as it was, forced him to examine who he was and what he was doing, and ultimately pushed him to create a new life for himself, one with more meaning and focus, one that is helping tens of thousands of others to lead a better life, one that he can't imagine changing.

A New Kind of Happiness

H'Sien Hayward grew up in Washington State's San Juan Islands, the daughter of hippies—she jokes that she learned to meditate before she learned how to walk. Her childhood was idyllic and unstructured. There were no rules. And that always gave her the confidence to pursue whatever she wanted to achieve, with little care for the obstacles. "My first-line assumption was always that I could do something," she says. She was athletic and a good student in high school—she would have been devastated with anything less than an A. She had lots of friends and dated the quarterback. She also played volleyball and basketball, ran track and cross-country. She was good enough that when she was sixteen she received a scholarship to compete in running for Hawaii Preparatory Academy, on the island of Hawaii.

On a trip to the beach with friends after her first year at her new school, the car that she was in hit another car on a winding mountain road. No one was seriously injured—except for Hayward, who suffered a severe spinal cord injury and was in a coma. Doctors told her parents to get to Hawaii within twenty-four hours if they wanted to see their daughter alive again. When her parents arrived, doctors told them that their daughter had suffered serious brain damage. They didn't think that she would be able to speak and might not even be able to breathe on her own. Ten days later Hayward woke from the coma and proved them wrong. Remarkably, she had no brain damage at all, but she was paralyzed from the chest down.

Her brother had died years earlier in an accident, so when their daughter woke from her coma, her parents were not sad about her paralysis. Instead they were overjoyed that she was alive at all. Given the alternative, this was a wonderful outcome. "They were so happy," says Hayward of her family. "The paralysis was secondary. She is alive and that's what counts."

After three weeks she was flown back to Seattle, where she spent another three months in a hospital. Hayward couldn't walk. And life in a wheelchair was not easy. She was used to being active and thought of herself as an athlete. Instead of competing on the athletic field, she learned to apply her competitive nature to her rehabilitation, challenging herself to relearn basic tasks that could help lead to greater independence, like putting on her socks and her shoes, and bathing. She was very lucky to have her parents' love and support and that of a boyfriend, too. "He was amazing," she says. "He helped me realize that I was beautiful and lovable and that what form I was in was irrelevant."

The five-year anniversary of the accident was perhaps the most trying time. Like most spinal cord injury survivors, Hayward held out hope that feeling and mobility would return to her legs. Though she was optimistic—a trait she gets from her mother—being in a wheelchair could be frustrating and simply hard. Bathing, getting dressed, getting places was slow. Sores could easily become infected because she couldn't feel them. Doctors who work with spinal cord injury patients have found that if nothing has improved in five years, the paralysis will be permanent. "It was sobering," she says. "For the first time I had to honestly look at the fact that I was going to spend the rest of my life in a wheelchair."

But she never let the disability deter her from her goals and interests. She excelled academically. She returned to her school in Hawaii after her accident and graduated with her class. She became interested in psychology and studied at Stanford, then went on to Harvard to get her Ph.D. She has become an outspoken advocate for the rights of people with disabilities. She has traveled the world—her goal is to visit fifty countries and she has already checked off more than forty from her list.

Hayward's experience with injury and paralysis has always informed her academic interests. And one thing that had bothered her for a long time is the research on happiness. Most people assume that people who use wheelchairs are unhappy or at least less happy than able-bodied people. It's not an unreasonable assumption. There are many things that able-bodied people can do that those in wheelchairs can't. Life is easier on two feet. And many of those in wheelchairs were once able-bodied. They have had that freedom and ease taken from them.

That assumption was bolstered decades ago by a well-known study coauthored by Ronnie Janoff-Bulman, who developed the assumptive-world theory that Tedeschi and Calhoun used for their model of post-traumatic growth. In a study published in 1978, Janoff-Bulman and her coauthors surveyed three groups: lottery winners, accident victims who were paralyzed, and a control group. They wanted to see who was happier. They contacted about twenty people in each group. The lottery winners won between $50,000 and $1 million.

They found that the accident victims had the lowest assessment of their present happiness of any of the groups. In the paper the researchers emphasized that the accident victims had the rosiest view of their past, something they called the nostalgia effect—they overestimated how happy they were before because their present circumstance was so dire.

Hayward was bothered by several things about the study. The samples were small—only about twenty or so people in each category. And those in the study had been injured very recently—only a month to a year before they were surveyed. A year is very little time to habituate to paralysis, as Hayward well knew. The subjects were all still in rehabilitation facilities. None had reintegrated into the world, nor had they likely even come to terms with their situation. And, she says, the results were often misinterpreted. The data from the original study show that the spinal cord injury victims were not just slightly less happy than the control group: the gap is quite large. One later study pointed out that the average person in the control group was happier than 78 percent of the crash victims.

Hayward thought that the study misrepresented her own experience and that of other spinal cord injury victims. She wanted to redo the study, this time bringing in a larger group. And she wanted the defining incident to have occurred much further in the past. There had been some subsequent research showing that those with spinal cord injuries like hers were as happy as or even more happy than those who had not been injured. But how did they compare to those who had the ultimate windfall—winning the lottery?

For her dissertation, Hayward increased the sample to fifty people for each group—control, lottery winners, and accident victims. The lottery winners had all won about a decade before. And all had won more than $1 million. The average winning was $6 million each— truly life-changing sums of money. Those with spinal cord injuries were about two decades removed from their accidents. Hayward surveyed all of the groups, including a control group, whose members had none of these experiences.

After so much time elapsed between the events—winning the lottery and being paralyzed—all of the groups had about the same level of happiness. They were essentially equal in terms of how they viewed their present happiness. The spinal cord injury group even scored slightly higher than the others on how much they enjoyed pleasurable daily activities. Hayward also found that the nostalgia effect disappeared and even that the accident victims had similar estimates of future happiness as the control group.

In other words, twenty years on, people all have about the same level of happiness, whether they had won the lottery, lost the use of their legs, or avoided either of these events. And, Hayward says, part of the reason for this is post-traumatic growth. She conducted another study of a larger group of people with spinal cord injuries for her dissertation, this time asking about their well-being, how much they earned, and how much meaning they had in their lives. She found no relationship between income and well-being. Instead the greatest factor in determining well-being was how much meaning these people had in their lives. And that sense of meaning, she says, is driving their happiness. "There was a lot more meaning in the lives of the accident survivors, a lot more meaning and a lot more growth, and that was the reason they looked happy," she says.

Psychologists have defined two types of happiness, both of which trace their origins to the ancient Greeks. Hedonic happiness is more closely associated with the pursuit of pleasure and the avoidance of pain—the pleasure one gets from eating an ice cream cone on a hot summer day, for example, or the enjoyable things that one can do with lottery winnings. This kind of happiness may lead to a lot of fun, but it is often fleeting and lacks greater purpose.

The other kind of happiness, eudaimonia, is deeper and related to pursuing personal growth and becoming a better person. This kind of happiness is much closer to the experience of those who report post-traumatic growth. Many lead lives steeped in meaning. They have a certain wisdom gained from experience and they value those who are closest to them. They are fulfilled, not simply having a good time.

Many of those who experience post-traumatic growth talk about just this kind of happiness. Luther Delp lost his life of hedonic happiness that day he was hit sitting at the stoplight on his motorcycle. All of the toys, the normal indulgences that all of us hope for, were stripped from him. But what he found instead was a new, much deeper, and more meaningful way of living his life. He has found a new, more valuable kind of happiness from helping others. The same is true for so many others. Karina Hollekim, who crashed from the sky in her wingsuit, finds value in herself and her work, inspiring others. So do Bob Carey and his wife, Linda Lancaster-Carey, who created the Tutu Project. That is at the core of growth for so many people, including Hayward. "The most important part of life for me is evolving as a person. And for me this opportunity to do that, to grow, has made me very happy," she says. "In my experience, as many if not more beautiful things came out of my accident as horrible things. Every day my heart is opened by people who will stop traffic to help me get across the street, push me up a hill, carry my groceries, or put me back in my chair when I've fallen. Every time I feel my heart opening."

Hayward is nearing the twentieth anniversary of her accident. She has been in her wheelchair longer than she had use of her legs. She has often thought about how the accident divided her life into two halves, and how her life after the accident was so different. The accident, the growth it sparked in her, has been a gift. "I've always been a cheerful person, but my happiness seems deeper now, more profound. My accident taught me that all of life can have beauty in it, both things that bring pleasure and those that bring pain. And it crystallized my life's work—I get to spend my days researching happiness, and am training to become a clinician," she says. "I love what I do, who I am, and can't imagine a better life."

And those changes show no sign of abating. Like Harriman, her life has been set on a new course and there is no wavering or turning back. "The way I look at life is that we are all working for personal growth; either we are conscious of it or not but we are bettering ourselves," she says. "Everyone is trying to get up the same stairs, but when you have something so difficult to challenge you, it's like you have been given an elevator to rise up several levels."

Trauma is not the debilitating experience that it seems to be. Those who survive traumatic experience have, by definition, survived. And given that they came so close to death, that they lost so many things they once took for granted, they understand on a much deeper level, in a much more informed way, what it means to be alive. Like few others they understand the gift and opportunity that exist in simply being alive. Hayward, like Harriman and so many others, is driven to do worthwhile and meaningful things with her life. And those pursuits bring each of them the kind of eudaimonic happiness that they rarely experienced before. It is part of why they do what they do and it is certainly part of why they will continue to live their lives according to the new course that was laid out for them the day they crossed paths with tragedy. They understand that trauma, for all of the misery it brings with it, also presents a remarkable opportunity.

Looking back on that day two decades ago when she chose to get into that car, to innocently catch a ride to the beach with her friends, the day that changed her life forever, Hayward says, "If I could go back twenty years and choose not to get in that car . . ." She pauses for just a beat, as if she's considering it again, thinking over what she lost that day and what she has gained since. ". . . I wouldn't change it," she says. "I would still do it."

ACKNOWLEDGMENTS

THROUGHOUT MY JOURNALISM CAREER, I HAVE HAD THE GOOD fortune to delve into many topics that fascinate me, to find and interview remarkable people and to tell their stories. But I can't think of any other reporting project that I have worked on that has been as meaningful and rewarding as the work that I have done on this book. I feel truly lucky to have been able to pursue this subject, to have met and spoken with each of these inspiring trauma survivors and to tell their stories. There are many, many people who helped to turn this idea into a book and allowed me to spend years immersed in the subject, and to them I am truly grateful.

Michelle Howry at Touchstone was willing to take a chance on the project and help shepherd it along. Without her belief in the idea and my ability to execute it, there would be no book at all. Nathaniel Jacks at InkWell Management was a constant source of wisdom and encouragement and a voice of calm when it was needed. Lisa Davis was a remarkable help, providing me with insights on storytelling techniques, helping to untangle my prose, and acting as a valued sounding board. Abner Kingman's keen eye and unrelenting demands for clear and well-organized writing helped to make the entire book a much more enjoyable read. Jon Bennett's and Lisa Shaw's hospitality, conversation, and ideas about the subject were invaluable.

A book like this is impossible to report and write without people who are willing to share their stories and their life's work. Richard Tedeschi and Lawrence Calhoun have been beyond patient, meeting with me in person, fielding phone calls and emails, and taking the time to teach me an incredible amount about their field and their life's work. Stephen Joseph and dozens of other researchers similarly took a great deal of time to speak with me, explain their papers, and point me to other experts and research. I appreciate and respect their work and their willingness to pursue this fascinating topic. Their decision to ignore the prevailing trends in psychology, to listen to their clients and to follow the findings of their own research regardless of the dominant point of view, is inspiring.

I owe each of the trauma survivors mentioned in the book (and many who were not) a deep debt of gratitude. They opened up to me, shared their life's most painful moments, their thoughts and insights and most personal stories. Each of them was open, honest, and thoughtful. They had spent so much time thinking about the events we discussed that all of them were articulate and insightful and a pleasure and a privilege to speak with. They made my job easy. I only wish that there was a place in the book for everyone whom I interviewed. I apologize to those who shared their remarkable stories with me who are not in the final draft.

And without talented editors willing to take a chance on my magazine stories about post-traumatic growth, there would also be no book. Vera Titunik at *The New York Times Magazine* championed the idea there for my article "Post-Traumatic Stress's Surprisingly Positive Flip Side." As always she pushed me to think in larger terms about the topic, to ask tough questions, and to write to my highest ability. Lea Goldman at *Marie Claire* saw the power of Karina Hollekim's story and helped me to turn around a richly reported tale of Hollekim's tragic accident and dramatic transformation in the article "Falling from Grace." I'd also like to thank Corinne Asturias, a talented editor who gave me my first journalism job, Kim Bernstein, a wonderful editor who is now a psychoanalyst, as well as Vera Titunik for recommending me for grants for the book.

And without the love and patience of my family, I would never have completed this project. Our sons, Sam and Zach, put up with plenty of nights and weekends without Daddy to play with. Thank you to my amazing wife, Kimberly Hamm, for her love, patience, counsel, and support.

A NOTE ON SOURCES

THIS BOOK IS BASED ON HUNDREDS OF INTERVIEWS—DISCUSSION
with dozens of trauma survivors and many of their friends and family members, many more psychologists, psychiatrists, social workers, and others who work with trauma survivors, study growth, PTSD, trauma and related topics. It is also based on hundreds of published studies and some that were not published. The sources who are named in the book and are referenced in any substantial way were given the opportunity to review the information attributed to them for the sake of accuracy. No source saw any information provided by another source and no source saw the entire book prior to its finalization. This was a helpful process that allowed me to ferret out errors and in some instances enabled me to follow up on ideas and deepen my reporting. Changes were made only for the sake of accuracy. In a few cases I have agreed to change a name or obscure an identity and those instances are clearly indicated in the text.

I originally wrote about Karin Hollekim, who appears in chapter 6, for *Marie Claire* magazine. That article is sourced in the Notes that follow. Much of the information about Hollekim and her life that is used here including many quotes from her and her friends and family members originally appeared in that article and I thank *Marie Claire* and my editor there for graciously allowing me to retell her story here. I also wrote about post-traumatic growth for *The New York Times Magazine* and some of the basic information about growth and a quote or two that originally appeared in that article also appear here. The article is also cited in the Notes.

NOTES

INTRODUCTION

x *"Nobody could believe what was going on":* When I visited Dora and other concentration camps with my father I taped our talks and taped while we walked around the camps. This quote is taken from those tapes. I also used this quote in an article that I wrote about reparations for slave laborers for *Metro* newspaper: Jim Rendon, "Cents of Outrage," *Metro*, March 23, 2000. http://www.metroactive.com/papers/metro/03.23.00 /cover/reparations-0012.html.

1. REVERSING PSYCHOLOGY

11 *In the opening of their first book:* Richard G. Tedeschi and Lawrence G. Calhoun, *Trauma and Transformation: Growing in the Aftermath of Suffering* (Thousand Oaks, CA: SAGE, 1995).

12 *One study they discovered:* William H. Sledge, James A. Boydstun, and Alton J. Rabe, "Self-Concept Changes Related to War Captivity," *Archives of General Psychiatry* 37, no. 4 (1980): 430–33, doi:10.1001/archpsyc .1980.01780170072008.

13 *In the fall of 1976, Sledge:* Ibid.

16 *interviewed more than six hundred trauma survivors:* I have written about post-traumatic growth for other publications, including "Post-Traumatic Stress's Surprisingly Positive Flip Side," *New York Times Magazine*, March

22, 2012. Though I spent much subsequent time with Tedeschi and Calhoun, some of the basic information about growth that appears here was gathered for that article.

16 *Their first paper detailing these positive changes:* Lawrence G. Calhoun and Richard G. Tedeschi, "Positive Aspects of Critical Life Problems: Recollections of Grief," *Omega* 20, no. 4 (1989–90): 265–72.

17 *Their Posttraumatic Growth Inventory:* Richard G. Tedeschi and Lawrence G. Calhoun, "The Posttraumatic Growth Inventory: Measuring the Positive Legacy of Trauma," *Journal of Traumatic Stress* 9, no. 3 (1996): 455–71, doi:10.1007/BF02103658.

17 *Half or more of all trauma survivors:* Ibid. and discussions with Richard Tedeschi.

17 *Growth, it turns out, is actually more common:* Jaimie L. Gradus, "Epidemiology of PTSD," PTSD: National Center for PTSD, December 22, 2014, http://www.ptsd.va.gov/professional/PTSD-overview/epidemiological -facts-ptsd.asp.

20 *Psychologists in China:* Yanbo Wang, Hongbiao Wang, Ji Wang, Jing Wu, and Xiaohong Liu, "Prevalence and Predictors of Posttraumatic Growth in Accidentally Injured Patients," *Journal of Clinical Psychology in Medical Settings* 20 (August 2012): 3–12, doi:10.1007/s10880-012-9315-2.

20 *Japan:* Kanako Taku, Arnie Cann, Richard G. Tedeschi, and Lawrence G. Calhoun, "Intrusive Versus Deliberate Rumination in Posttraumatic Growth Across US and Japanese Samples," *Anxiety, Stress & Coping* 22 (March 2009): 129–36, doi:10.1080/10615800802082296.

20 *Turkey:* Ayse Nuray Karanci et al., "Personality, Posttraumatic Stress, and Trauma Type: Factors Contributing to Posttraumatic Growth and Its Domains in a Turkish Community Sample," *European Journal of Psychotraumatology* 3 (June 2012), doi:10.3402/ejpt.v3i0.17303.

20 *Iran:* Farah Lotfi-Kashani, Shahram Vaziri, Mohammad Esmaeil Akbari, Nahid Kazemi-Zanjani, and Leila Shamkoeyan, "Predicting Post Traumatic Growth Based upon Self-Efficacy and Perceived Social Support in Cancer Patients," *Iranian Journal of Cancer Prevention* 7, no. 3 (2014): 115–23, http://www.researchgate.net/journal/2008-2401_Iranian_Journal _of_Cancer_Prevention.

20 *Italy:* Chiara Ruini, Francesca Vescovelli, and Elisa Albieri, "Post-Traumatic Growth in Breast Cancer Survivors: New Insights into Its Re-

lationships with Well-Being and Distress," *Journal of Clinical Psychology in Medical Settings* 20, no. 3 (2013): 383–91, doi:10.1007/s10880-012 -9340-1.

20 *England:* Trevor Powell, Rachael Gilson, and Christine Collin, "TBI 13 Years On: Factors Associated with Post-Traumatic Growth," *Disability and Rehabilitation* 34 (August 2012): 1461–67, doi:10.3109/09638288 .2011.644384.

20 *Australia:* J. E. Shakespeare-Finch, S. G. Smith, K. M. Gow, G. Embelton, and L. Baird, "The Prevalence of Post-Traumatic Growth in Emergency Ambulance Personnel," *Traumatology* 9 (March 2003): 58–71, doi:10.1177/153476560300900104.

20 *Israel:* Sharon Dekel, Tsachi Ein-Dor, and Zahava Solomon, "Posttraumatic Growth and Posttraumatic Distress: A Longitudinal Study," *Psychological Trauma* 4 (January 2012): 94–101, doi:10.1037/a0021865.

21 *cancer survivors and their spouses:* Tzipi Weiss, "Posttraumatic Growth in Women with Breast Cancer and Their Husbands: An Intersubjective Validation Study," *Journal of Psychosocial Oncology* 20, no. 21 (2002): 65–80, doi:10.1300/J077v20n02_04.

21 *prisoners of war:* Dekel, "Posttraumatic Growth and Posttrauamtic Distress."

21 *immigrants:* Roni Berger and Tzipi Weiss, "Posttraumatic Growth in Latina Immigrants," *Journal of Immigrant & Refugee Studies* 4, no. 3 (2006): 55–72, doi:10.1300/J500v04n03_03.

21 *survivors of natural disaster:* Johan Siqveland, Gertrud Sofie Hafstad, and Richard G. Tedeschi, "Posttraumatic Growth in Parents After a Natural Disaster," *Journal of Loss and Trauma* 17, no. 6 (2012): 536–44, doi:10.1 080/15325024.2012.678778.

2. THE PSYCHIATRIST IN THE DEATH CAMP

23 *In 1942, Viktor Frankl:* Throughout this chapter the account of Viktor E. Frankl's time in concentration camps and the psychological understanding that he gained from that experience is taken from his book *Man's Search for Meaning,* trans. Ilse Lasch (1946; reprint, Boston: Beacon Press, 2006). I will cite page numbers for specific quotes from the book.

23 *"Under the influence of a world":* Ibid., p. 50.

24 *"He who has a* why *to live can bear with almost any* how": Ibid., p. 104.

25 *"suffering is not always a pathological phenomenon"*: Ibid., p. 102.

26 *new perspective on life:* Information on the humanistic psychologists comes from an interview with Louis Hoffman, who holds the Existential, Humanistic, and Transpersonal Psychology Specialization Chair at Saybrook University.

26 *it was not even recognized as a diagnosis until 1980:* Matthew J. Friedman, "PTSD History and Overview," U.S. Department of Veterans Affairs website, http://www.ptsd.va.gov/professional/PTSD-overview/ptsd -overview.asp.

27 *75 percent of people will experience a traumatic event in their lifetime:* Naomi Breslau and Ronald C. Kessler, "The Stressor Criterion in *DSM– IV* Posttraumatic Stress Disorder: An Empirical Investigation," *Biological Psychiatry* 50, no. 9 (November 1, 2001).

27 *In the 1980s, Stephen Joseph:* Accounts of Stephen Joseph's work are taken from interviews with him and from his book *What Doesn't Kill Us: The New Psychology of Posttraumatic Growth* (New York: Basic Books, 2011).

29 *In the 1990s, Martin Seligman:* Accounts of Martin Seligman and his work are based on an interview with him, as well as observations of his Comprehensive Soldier Fitness course conducted for the U.S. Army in April 2011; from watching his talk at the 92nd Street Y in New York City on April 4, 2011; and from his book *Flourish: A Visionary New Understanding of Happiness and Well-Being* (New York: Free Press, 2011).

31 *people are unreliable:* Patricia Frazier, Howard Tennen, Margaret Gavian, Crystal Park, Patricia Tomich, and Ty Tashiro, "Does Self-Reported Posttraumatic Growth Reflect Genuine Positive Change?" *Psychological Science* 20, no. 7 (July 2009); Howard Tennen and Glenn Affleck, "Assessing Positive Life Change: In Search of Meticulous Methods," in *Medical Illness and Positive Life Change: Can Crisis Lead to Personal Transformation?* ed. Crystal L. Park, Suzanne C. Lechner, Michael H. Antoni, and Annette L. Stanton (Washington, DC: APA Press, 2009), pp. 31–49.

32 *positive changes reported by the trauma survivors:* Jane Shakespeare-Finch and Tracey Enders, "Corroborating Evidence of Posttraumatic Growth," *Journal of Traumatic Stress* 21, no. 4 (August 1, 2008).

33 *influenced by the culture:* Tennen and Affleck, "Assessing Positive Life Change"; Katie Splevins, Keren Cohe, Jake Bowley, and Stephen Joseph,

"Theories of Posttraumatic Growth: Cross-Cultural Perspectives," *Journal of Loss and Trauma* 16, no. 3 (2010).

35 *later as president:* The preceding account of Theodore Roosevelt's life was taken largely from the biography by Edmund Morris, *The Rise of Theodore Roosevelt* (New York: Random House, 2010).

35 *Christopher Nolan, who directed the 2005 film:* Steven Smith, *Batman Unmasked: The Psychology of the Dark Knight,* 2008, television documentary, History Channel.

37 *other populations around the world:* All of the studies mentioned in this paragraph can be found in Tzipi Weiss and Roni Berger, *Posttraumatic Growth and Culturally Competent Practice: Lessons Learned from Around the Globe* (Hoboken, NJ: Wiley, 2010).

3. THAT WAS TRAUMATIC?

38 *In April 1968, Max Cleland:* Accounts of Max Cleland's life are taken from interviews I conducted with him and from Max Cleland with Ben Raines, *Heart of a Patriot: How I Found the Courage to Survive Vietnam, Walter Reed and Karl Rove* (New York: Simon & Schuster, 2009).

40 *During an event like this:* The account of how the brain functions in a life-threatening situation was reported from Joseph Le Doux, *Anxious: Using the Brain to Understand and Treat Fear and Anxiety* (New York: Viking, 2015), pp. 31, 97, 209–11, 216.

42 *he and his coauthors devised an experiment:* Chess Stetson, Matthew P. Fiesta, and David M. Eagleman, "Does Time Really Slow Down During a Frightening Event?" *PloS One* (December 12, 2007).

44 *Goosens found that the body releases ghrelin:* R. M. Meyer, A. Burgos-Robles, E. Liu, S. S. Correia, and K. A. Goosens, "A Ghrelin–Growth Hormone Axis Drives Stress-Induced Vulnerability to Enhanced Fear," *Molecular Psychiatry* 19, no. 12 (December 2014), published online October 2013.

47 *Most people who survive a traumatic event:* Le Doux, *Anxious*, pp. 109–11.

47 *Le Doux, in his 1996 book:* Le Doux, *The Emotional Brain: The Mysterious Underpinnings of Emotional Life* (New York: Simon & Schuster, 1996), p. 257.

48 *Severe stress has even been:* Le Doux, *The Emotional Brain*, pp. 242–43.

49 *"In my mind I replayed the grenade explosion":* Cleland and Raines, *Heart of a Patriot,* pp. 62–63.

50 *Shvil replicated a well-known Harvard experiment:* Mohammed R. Milad et al., "Neurobiological Basis of Failure to Recall Extinction Memory in Posttraumatic Stress Disorder," *Biological Psychiatry* 66, no. 12 (2009).

52 *what kind of trauma could trigger the disorder:* Friedman, "PTSD History and Overview."

52 *About 20 percent of those who simply happened to live south of Canal Street:* Sandro Galea et al., "Psychological Sequelae of the September 11 Terrorist Attacks in New York City," *New England Journal of Medicine* 346, no. 14 (March 28, 2002).

53 *recorded in cancer survivors and in their spouses as well:* Tzipi Weiss, "Correlates of Posttraumatic Growth in Husbands of Breast Cancer Survivors," *Psycho-Oncology* 13, no. 4 (April 2004).

53 *9 percent of women exhibited the symptoms of full-blown PTSD following childbirth:* Cheryl Tatano Beck, Robert K. Gable, Carol Sakala, and Eugene R. Declercq, "Posttraumatic Stress Disorder in New Mothers: Results from a Two-Stage U.S. National Survey," *Birth* 38 (September 2011). The findings of this study are on the high end of many estimates that place the prevalence of PTSD among new mothers between 2 percent and 9 percent.

53 *more than half of the women surveyed after childbirth:* Alexandra Sawyer and Susan Ayers, "Post Traumatic Growth in Women After Childbirth," *Psychology and Health* (April 2009).

54 *She decided to study the Madoff victims:* Audrey Freshman, "Financial Disaster as a Risk Factor for Posttraumatic Stress Disorder: Internet Survey of Trauma in Victims of the Madoff Ponzi Scheme," *Health and Social Work* 37, no. 1 (July 2012).

55 *those with less severe trauma report less growth:* The entire phenomenon discussed here, the inverted U, is discussed and well sourced in Joseph, *What Doesn't Kill Us.* See his notes to chapter 4, number 35, on p. 227 for many specific studies.

55 *spouses of former Israeli prisoners of war:* Rachel Dekel, "Posttraumatic Distress and Growth Among Wives of Prisoners of War: The Contribution of Husbands' Posttraumatic Stress Disorder and Wives' Own Attachment," *American Journal of Orthopsychiatry* 77, no. 3 (July 2007).

56 *A study published in 2012 by researchers in Israel:* Sharon Dekel, Tsachi Ein-Dor, and Zahava Solomon, "Posttraumatic Growth and Posttraumatic Distress: A Longitudinal Study," *Psychological Trauma* 4, no. 1 (January 2012).

57 *and the worse they were treated:* Sledge, "Self-Concept Changes."

58 *brain images can be used as a diagnostic tool with about 90 percent accuracy:* A. P. Georgopoulos et al., "The Synchronous Neural Interactions Test as a Functional Neuromarker for Post-Traumatic Stress Disorder (PTSD): A Robust Classification Method Based on the Bootstrap," *Journal of Neural Engineering* 7, no. 1 (February 2010).

4. TELLING A NEW STORY

63 *Just a few years ago, Mullins was one of those students:* The account of Shane Mullins's story is from phone and in-person interviews with Mullins and his mother, Rose, and from attending his talk at Galway Technical Institute. Mullins asked that readers look for D'mess on Facebook and Twitter for more information.

70 *beliefs that are incompatible with traumatic experience:* Though Janoff-Bulman says she no longer gives interviews about her work on trauma and shattered assumptions (she would not speak with me despite my requests for an interview), the following paper describes her ideas: Ronnie Janoff-Bulman, "Assumptive Worlds and the Stress of Traumatic Events: Applications of the Schema Construct," *Social Cognition* 7 no. 2 (1989). Her book is also a great resource: Ronnie Janoff-Bulman, *Shattered Assumptions: Towards a New Psychology of Trauma* (New York: Free Press, 2002).

70 *three British researchers:* Wendy Middleton, Peter Harris, and Mark Surman, "Give 'Em Enough Rope: Perception of Health and Safety Risks in Bungee Jumpers," *Journal of Social and Clinical Psychology* 15, no. 1 (1996).

72 *theories advanced by developmental psychologist Jean Piaget:* Joseph uses this example in his book *What Doesn't Kill Us.* I used his book and interviews with him for this example.

73 *the 1995 historical epic* Braveheart: Mel Gibson, dir., *Braveheart*, Paramount Pictures, 1995.

74 *One, by LIU Post assistant professor Tzipi Weiss:* Tzipi Weiss, "Correlates of Posttraumatic Growth in Married Breast Cancer Survivors," *Journal of Social and Clinical Psychology* 23, no. 5 (2004).

74 *Weiss knows firsthand just how much role models can help:* Tzipi Weiss, "A Researcher's Personal Narrative: Positive Emotions, Mythical Thinking, and Posttraumatic Growth," *Traumatology* 11, no. 4 (December 2005).

76 *For a paper published in 2013, Suzanne Danhauer:* Suzanne C. Danhauer et al., "A Longitudinal Investigation of Posttraumatic Growth in Adult Patients Undergoing Treatment for Acute Leukemia," *Journal of Clinical Psychology in Medical Settings* 20, no. 1 (March 2013).

5. RELYING ON OTHERS

88 *A study of mothers in New Orleans:* Sarah R. Lowe, Christian S. Chan, and Jean E. Rhodes, "Pre-Hurricane Perceived Social Support Protects Against Psychological Distress: A Longitudinal Analysis of Low-Income Mothers," *Journal of Consulting and Clinical Psychology* 78, no. 4 (2010).

88 *A study of those affected by the terrorist attacks in New York City:* S. E. Perlman et al., "Short-Term and Medium-Term Health Effects of 9/11," *Lancet* 378, no. 9794 (September 2011).

88 *One study of women traumatized by the war in Bosnia:* Miro Klaric et al., "Social Support and PTSD Symptoms in War-Traumatized Women in Bosnia and Herzegovina," *Psychiatria Danubina* 20, no. 4 (2008).

90 *best predictor of post-traumatic growth was the level of social support:* Shira Maguen, Dawne S. Vogt, Lynda A. King, Daniel W. King, and Brett Litz, "Posttraumatic Growth Among Gulf War I Veterans: The Predictive Role of Deployment-Related Experiences and Background Characteristics," *Journal of Loss and Trauma* 11, no. 5 (2006).

90 *similar results with cancer patients:* Meghan H. McDonough, Catherine M. Sabisto, and Carsten Wrosch, "Predicting Changes in Posttraumatic Growth and Subjective Well-Being Among Breast Cancer Survivors: The Role of Social Support and Stress," *Psycho-Oncology* 23, no. 1 (January 2014).

90 *traumatic brain injury patients:* Trevor Powell, Rachael Gilson, and Christine Collin, "TBI 13 Years On: Factors Associated with Post-Traumatic Growth," *Disability and Rehabilitation* 34 (August 2012): 1461–67, doi: 10.3109/09638288.2011.644384.

90 *survivors of natural disasters:* A. Nuray Karanci and Acarturk, "Post-Traumatic Growth Among Marmara Earthquake Survivors Involved in

Disaster Preparedness as Volunteers," *Traumatology* 11, no. 4 (December 2005).

91 *Outgoing people are more likely to share:* Ibid.; Ayse Nuray Karanci et al., "Personality, Posttraumatic Stress, and Trauma Type: Factors Contributing to Posttraumatic Growth and Its Domains in a Turkish Community Sample," *European Journal of Psychotraumatology* 3 (2012).

99 *exercises to foster feelings of gratitude:* Martin E. P. Seligman, *Flourish: A Visionary New Understanding of Happiness and Well-Being* (New York: Free Press, 2011), pp. 30–31.

100 *gratitude was strongly linked to better health and psychological well-being:* Chiara Ruini and Francesca Vescovelli, "The Role of Gratitude in Breast Cancer: Its Relationships with Post-Traumatic Growth, Psychological Well-Being and Distress," *Journal of Happiness Studies* 4, no. 1 (March 2013).

6. EXPRESSING YOURSELF

103 *In August 2006, Karina Hollekim:* I originally wrote about Karina Hollekim for *Marie Claire* magazine: Jim Rendon, "Falling Towards Grace," *Marie Claire*, February 2013, http://www.marieclaire.com/politics/news/a7413/falling-toward-grace/. I have used my notes and additional interviews and email correspondence to rewrite much of this section on Hollekim; however, her life story is the same and the article and the chapter in the book both focus on how her skydiving accident transformed her life, so much of the basic structure of her story, the details of her life and quotes from her, her friends, and family are reproduced here with the permission of *Marie Claire.*

111 *One study conducted on breast cancer survivors and their spouses:* Sharon Manne, Jamie Ostroff, Gary Winkel, Lori Goldstein, Kevin Fox, and Generosa Grana, "Posttraumatic Growth After Breast Cancer: Patient, Partner, and Couple Perspectives," *Psychosomatic Medicine* 66, no. 3 (May 2004).

111 *women grew more, and more often, than male trauma survivors:* Tanya Vishnevsky, Arnie Cann, Lawrence G. Calhoun, Richard G. Tedeschi, and George J. Demakis, "Gender Differences in Self-Reported Posttraumatic Growth: A Meta-Analysis," *Psychology of Women Quarterly* 34, no. 1 (March 2010).

111 *but also according to some research:* Carolyn A. Liebler and Gary D. Sandefur, "Gender Differences in the Exchange of Social Support with Friends, Neighbors, and Co-Workers at Midlife," *Social Science Research* 31, no. 3 (2002); Anita P. Barbee et al., "Effects of Gender-Role Expectations on the Social Support Process," *Journal of Social Issues* 49, no. 3 (1993).

114 *Pennebaker devised an experiment:* James W. Pennebaker and Sandra Beall, "Confronting a Traumatic Event: Toward an Understanding of Inhibition and Disease," *Journal of Abnormal Psychology* 95 no. 3 (August 1986).

114 *That was the beginning of a long line of studies:* The following paper includes a review of much of the literature on expressive writing, including many of Pennebaker's own studies: James W. Pennebaker and Cindy K. Chung, "Expressive Writing and Its Links to Mental and Physical Health," in H. S. Friedman, ed., *Oxford Handbook of Health Psychology* (New York: Oxford University Press, in press). Pennebaker's books on the subject include *Opening Up: The Healing Power of Expressing Emotion* (New York: Guilford Press, 1990) and *Writing to Heal: A Guided Journal for Recovering from Trauma & Emotional Upheaval* (Oakland, CA: Harbinger Press, 2004).

115 *For one study published in 1995:* Keith J. Petrie, Roger Booth, James W. Pennebaker, Kathryn P. Davison, and Mark Thomas, "Disclosure of Trauma and Immune Response to Hepatitis B Vaccination Program," *Journal of Consulting and Clinical Psychology* 63, no. 5 (September 1995).

115 *One review of studies on expressive writing:* Joshua M. Smyth, "Written Emotional Expression: Effect Sizes, Outcome Types, and Moderating Variables," *Journal of Consulting and Clinical Psychology* 66, no. 1 (February 1998).

115 *subsequent meta-analyses have generally agreed:* Pasquale G. Frisina, Joan C. Borod, and Stephen J. Lepore, "A Meta-Analysis of the Effects of Written Emotional Disclosure on the Health Outcomes of Clinical Populations," *Journal of Nervous and Mental Disease* 192, no. 9 (September 2004). Also see Pennebaker and Chung, "Expressive Writing and Its Links to Mental and Physical Health."

115 *expressive writing reduced blood pressure:* Kimberly M. Beckwith McGuire, Melanie A. Greenberg, and Richard Gevirtz, "Autonomic Effects of Expressive Writing in Individuals with Elevated Blood Pressure," *Journal of Health Psychology* 10, no. 2 (April 2005).

115 *showed an improvement in their grades:* Mark A. Lumley and Kimberly M. Provenzano, "Stress Management Through Written Emotional Disclosure Improves Academic Performance Among College Students with Physical Symptoms," *Journal of Educational Psychology* 95, no. 3 (September 2003).

115 *helped job seekers get hired more quickly:* Stefanie P. Spera, Eric D. Buhrfeind, and James W. Pennebaker, "Expressive Writing and Coping with Job Loss," *Academy of Management Journal* 37, no. 3 (1994).

115 *Even expressive writing for two minutes two days in a row:* Chad M. Burton and Laura A. King, "Effects of (Very) Brief Writing on Health: The Two-Minute Miracle," *British Journal of Health Psychology* 13, no. 1 (February 2008).

116 *using bodily movement:* Anne M. Krantz and James W. Pennebaker, "Expressive Dance, Writing, Trauma, and Health: When Words Have a Body," in Ileen A. Serlin, ed., *Whole Person Healthcare*, vol. 3, *The Arts and Health* (Westport, CT: Praeger, 2007), pp. 201–29.

116 *organized way is more beneficial than doing it in a disorganized way:* Pennebaker and Chung, "Expressive Writing and Its Links to Mental and Physical Health."

117 *writing demands such organization:* Ibid.

117 *In a study Smyth conducted:* Joshua M. Smyth, "Expressive Writing and Post-Traumatic Stress Disorder: Effects on Trauma Symptoms, Mood States, and Cortisol Reactivity," *British Journal of Health Psychology* 13, no. 1 (February 2008).

7. LOOKING FOR THE POSITIVE

129 *the role of positive emotion in health:* Pennebaker and Chung, "Expressive Writing and Its Links to Mental and Physical Health."

131 *a review of thirty-nine separate studies:* P. Alex Linley and Stephen Joseph, "Positive Change Following Trauma and Adversity: A Review," *Journal of Traumatic Stress* 17, no. 1 (February 2004).

132 *One study conducted on cancer survivors in China:* Samuel Ho et al., "The Roles of Hope and Optimism on Posttraumatic Growth in Oral Cavity Cancer Patients," *Oral Oncology* 47, no. 2 (February 2011).

132 *small relationship between optimism and growth:* Lucy Bostock, Alia I. Sheikh, and Stephen Barton, "Posttraumatic Growth and Optimism in Health-Related Trauma: A Systematic Review," *Journal of Clinical Psychology in Medical Settings* 16, no. 4 (December 2009).

136 *A study of forty-one cancer patients conducted in Italy:* Marta Scrignaro, Sandro Barni, and Maria Elena Magrin, "The Combined Contribution of Social Support and Coping Strategies in Predicting Post-Traumatic Growth: A Longitudinal Study on Cancer Patients," *Psycho-Oncology* 20, no. 8 (August 2011).

8. FINDING MEANING IN FAITH

142 *the religion's most basic story, about the Buddha's origin:* The descriptions of the life of Buddha and the Mahabharata are from an interview and email correspondence with Daniel Veidlinger, an associate professor at California State University, Chico who specializes in Eastern religions.

146 *something Pargament calls religious coping:* Kenneth I. Pargament, Harold G. Koenig, and Lisa M. Perez, "The Many Methods of Religious Coping: Development and Initial Validation of the RCOPE," *Journal of Clinical Psychology* 56, no. 4 (April 2000).

148 *Feigelman studied 426 parents:* William Feigelman, John R. Jordan, and Bernard S. Gorman, "Personal Growth After a Suicide Loss: Cross-Sectional Findings Suggest Growth After Loss May Be Associated with Better Mental Health Among Survivors," *Omega* 53, no. 9 (2009).

148 *One study published in 2006:* Suzanne C. Lechner, Charles S. Carver, Michael H. Antoni, Kathryn E. Weaver, and Kristin M. Phillips, "Curvilinear Associations Between Benefit Finding and Psychosocial Adjustment to Breast Cancer," *Journal of Consulting and Clinical Psychology* 74, no. 5 (October 2006).

148 *One large review of 103 studies of post-traumatic growth:* Gabriele Prati and Luca Pietrantoni, "Optimism, Social Support, and Coping Strategies as Factors Contributing to Posttraumatic Growth: A Meta-Analysis," *Journal of Loss and Trauma* 14, no. 5 (2009).

151 *surveyed and interviewed sixty-one breast cancer patients:* Avinash Thombre, Allen C. Sherman, and Stephanie Simonton, "Posttraumatic Growth Among Cancer Patients in India," *Journal of Behavioral Medicine* 33, no. 1 (February 2010).

152 *Thombre conducted another study in India of fifty-eight caregivers:* Avinash Thombre, Allen C. Sherman, and Stephanie Simonton, "Religious Coping and Posttraumatic Growth Among Family Caregivers of Cancer Patients in India," *Journal of Psychosocial Oncology* 28, no. 2 (2010).

9. OPENING UP TO NEW EXPERIENCES

156 *In 2012, they self-published a book:* Bob Carey, *Ballerina*, self-published, 2012.

161 *reducing the length of hospital stays:* Heather L. Stuckey and Jeremy Nobel, "The Connection Between Art, Healing, and Public Health: A Review of Current Literature," *American Journal of Public Health* 100, no. 2 (February 2010).

161 *boost quality of life and decrease depression and anxiety:* Kristina Geue, Heide Goetze, Marianne Buttstaedt, Evelyn Kleinert, Diana Richter, and Susanne Singer, "An Overview of Art Therapy Interventions for Cancer Patients and the Results of Research," *Complementary Therapies in Medicine* 18, nos. 3–4 (June–August 2010).

161 *flow, an intense concentration that merges both action and awareness:* I learned a lot about many of the basic concepts of art therapy from papers by Marie J. Forgeard, who is quoted later in this chapter. Many of the studies I cite I discovered from reading her papers. The following book chapter was particularly helpful: Marie J. C. Forgeard, Anne C. Mecklenburg, Justin J. Lacasse, and Eranda Jayawickreme, "Bringing the Whole Universe to Order: Creativity, Healing, and Posttraumatic Growth," in James C. Kauffman, ed., *Creativity and Mental Illness* (Cambridge: Cambridge University Press, 2014), pp. 321–42.

165 *is openness to new experience:* Ayse Nuray Karanci et al., "Personality, Posttraumatic Stress, and Trauma Type: Factors Contributing to Posttraumatic Growth and Its Domains in a Turkish Community Sample," *European Journal of Psychotraumatology* 3 (2012).

165 *often have an interest in, and appreciation for, art:* Robert R. McCrae and Paul T. Costa, "Validation of the Five-Factor Model of Personality Across Instruments and Observers," *Journal of Personality and Social Psychology* 52, no. 1 (January 1987).

166 *a book about illness and creativity:* Tobi Zausner, *When Walls Become Doorways: Creativity and the Transforming Illness* (New York: Harmony Books, 2006).

167 *Henri Matisse, she points out, had no interest in art:* The account of Matisse's life and illnesses is taken from Zausner, *When Walls Become Doorways,* and from an interview with Zausner.

168 *Maya Angelou, for example, was raped by her mother's boyfriend:* Joanne M. Braxton, *Maya Angelou's I Know Why the Caged Bird Sings: A Casebook* (Oxford: Oxford University Press, 1999), p. 121.

168 *Frida Kahlo survived polio:* Hayden Herrera, *Frida: A Biography of Frida Kahlo* (New York: Harper & Row, 1983).

168 *Francis Ford Coppola also had polio:* Biography available via the Academy of Motion Picture Arts and Sciences website, http://www.oscars.org /governors-awards/2010/francis-ford-coppola.

169 *One study found that writers:* Dean Keith Simonton, *Greatness: Who Makes History and Why* (New York: Guilford Press, 1994).

169 *Forgeard wanted to examine:* Marie J. C. Forgeard, "Perceiving Benefits After Adversity: The Relationship Between Self-Reported Posttraumatic Growth and Creativity," *Psychology of Aesthetics, Creativity, and the Arts* 7, no. 3 (2013).

169 *In a separate study:* Marie Forgeard, "The Role of Openness to Experience in Growth Through Adversity," paper presented at The Most Consequential Trait? New Directions in Openness to Experience Research, symposium chaired by Eranda Jayawickreme and held at the Biennial Conference of the Association for Research in Personality, Charlotte, North Carolina, June 2013.

10. RACING BOATS AND CLIMBING MOUNTAINS

177 *For a study published in 2007:* Catherine M. Sabiston, Meghan H. McDonough, and Peter R. E. Crocker, "Psychosocial Experiences of Breast Cancer Survivors Involved in a Dragon Boat Program: Exploring Links to Positive Psychological Growth," *Journal of Sport & Exercise Psychology* 29, no. 4 (August 2007).

178 *In 2011 McDonough published another small study:* Meghan H. McDonough, Catherine M. Sabiston, and Sarah Ullrich-French, "The Development of Social Relationships, Social Support, and Posttraumatic Growth in a Dragon Boating Team for Breast Cancer Survivors," *Journal of Sport & Exercise Psychology* 33, no. 5 (October 2011).

180 *D. J. Skelton, a young lieutenant:* The account of D. J. Skelton's life and injuries in Iraq are from interviews with Skelton and from Bill Murphy Jr., "A warrior unbowed: Captain's wounds will never heal, but he's a better man because of them," *Stars and Stripes,* April 26, 2012 http://www .stripes.com/a-warrior-unbowed-captain-s-wounds-will-never-heal-but -he-s-a-better-man-because-of-them-1.175632.

183 *One review of nearly a dozen studies of combat veterans participating in sports:* Nick Caddick and Brett Smith, "The Impact of Sport and Physical Activity on the Well-Being of Combat Veterans: A Systematic Review," *Psychology of Sport and Exercise* 15, no. 1 (January 2014).

183 *A study of Paralympic athletes:* Jennifer J. Crawford, Amy M. Gayman, and Jill Tracey, "An Examination of Post-Traumatic Growth in Canadian and American ParaSport Athletes with Acquired Spinal Cord Injury," *Psychology of Sport and Exercise* 15, no. 4 (July 2014).

184 *In the study, published in 2008:* Kate Hefferon, Madeleine Grealy, and Nanette Mutrie, "The Perceived Influence of an Exercise Class Intervention on the Process and Outcomes of Post-Traumatic Growth," *Mental Health and Physical Activity* 1, no. 1 (June 2008).

184 *Her 2008 study found:* Ibid.

11. BONDING WITH THOSE WHO GET IT

197 *A 2008 review of studies of those using online support groups:* Azy Barak, Meyran Boniel-Nissim, and John Suler, "Fostering Empowerment in Online Support Groups," *Computers in Human Behavior* 24, no. 9 (September 2008).

197 *Another study of those with breast cancer and other ailments:* Cornelia F. van Uden-Kraan et al., "Empowering Processes and Outcomes of Participation in Online Support Groups for Patients with Breast Cancer, Arthritis, or Fibromyalgia," *Qualitative Health Research* 18, no. 3 (March 2008).

197 *A 2012 study of Iraq and Afghanistan War veterans:* Benjamin W. Van Voorhees, Jackie Gollan, and Joshua Fogel, "Pilot Study of Internet-Based Early Intervention for Combat-Related Mental Distress," *Journal of Rehabilitation Research & Development* 49, no. 8 (2012).

202 *Those with strong social networks report less PTSD and depression:* Sarah R. Lowe, Christian S. Chan, and Jean E. Rhodes, "Pre-Hurricane Perceived

Social Support Protects Against Psychological Distress: A Longitudinal Analysis of Low-Income Mothers," *Journal of Consulting and Clinical Psychology* 78, no. 4 (2010); S. E. Perlman et al., "Short-Term and Medium-Term Health Effects of 9/11," *Lancet* 378, no. 9794 (September 2011); Miro Klaric et al., "Social Support and PTSD Symptoms in War-Traumatized Women," *Psychiatria Danubina* 20, no. 4 (2008).

202 *And social support has been linked to growth:* Shira Maguen, Dawne S. Vogt, Lynda A. King, Daniel W. King, and Brett Litz, "Posttraumatic Growth Among Gulf War I Veterans: The Predictive Role of Deployment-Related Experiences and Background Characteristics," *Journal of Loss and Trauma* 11, no. 5 (2006).

203 *Powell conducted a study, published in 2012:* Trevor Powell, Rachael Gilson, and Christine Collin, "TBI 13 Years On: Factors Associated with Post-Traumatic Growth," *Disability and Rehabilitation* 34 (August 2012): 1461–67, doi:10.3109/09638288.2011.644384.

204 *survival rate for those with neuroblastoma in 1990 and the day that Hazen was diagnosed:* John M. Maris, Michael D. Hogarty, Rochelle Bagatell, Susan L. Cohn, "Neuroblastoma," *Lancet* (June 23, 2007) 369:21106-2120, and from conversations that Kennedy had with several pediatric oncologists.

12. MANAGING DISTRESS AND LEARNING TO GROW

211 *the response to traumatic events is often so overwhelming:* The information about how people commonly respond to trauma is taken in part from Stephanie D. Nelson, "The Posttraumatic Growth Path: An Emerging Model for Prevention and Treatment of Trauma-Related Behavioral Health Conditions," *Journal of Psychotherapy Integration* 21, no. 1 (March 2011), and confirmed with other psychologists familiar with trauma.

214 *one study by researchers at the University of Miami:* Michael H. Antoni et al., "Cognitive-Behavioral Stress Management Intervention Decreases the Prevalence of Depression and Enhances Benefit Finding Among Women Under Treatment for Early-Stage Breast Cancer," *Health Psychology* 20, no. 1 (January 2001).

222 *the book that she wrote detailing the therapeutic process:* Stephanie Dawn Nelson, *The Growth Path: Transforming Your Trauma,* unpublished manuscript.

13. FULFILLMENT VS. HAPPINESS

236 *growth in those who had been discharged:* Jenni Silva, Tamara Ownsworth, Cassandra Shields, and Jennifer Fleming, "Enhanced Appreciation of Life Following Acquired Brain Injury: Post-Traumatic Growth at 6 Months Postdischarge," *Brain Impairment* 12, no. 2 (September 2011).

236 *another at 7 months after:* Trevor Powell, Abigail Ekin-Wood, and Christine Collin, "Post-Traumatic Growth After Head Injury: A Long-Term Follow-Up," *Brain Injury* 21, no. 1 (February 2007).

236 *averaging 32 months after their injury:* Berit Gangstad, Paul Norman, and Jane Barton, "Cognitive Processing and Post-Traumatic Growth After Stroke," *Rehabilitation Psychology* 54, no. 1 (February 2009).

236 *She conducted her own study:* Carol Rogan, Dónal G. Fortune, and Garry Prentice, "Post-Traumatic Growth, Illness Perceptions, and Coping in People with Acquired Brain Injury," *Neuropsychological Rehabilitation* 23, no. 5 (May 2013).

236 *brain injuries an average of thirteen years after the initial injury:* Powell, Gilson, and Collin, "TBI 13 Years On."

241 *In a study published in 1978:* Philip Brickman, Dan Coates, Ronnie Janoff-Bulman, "Lottery Winners and Accident Victims: Is Happiness Relative?" *Journal of Personality and Social Psychology* 36, no. 8 (1978).

242 *One later study:* Ed Diener, Richard E. Lucas, and Christie Napa Scollon, "Beyond the Hedonic Treadmill: Revising the Adaptation Theory of Well-Being," *American Psychologist* 61, no. 4 (May–June 2006).

242 *those with spinal cord injuries like hers were as happy:* Richard Schulz and Susan Decker, "Long-Term Adjustment to Physical Disability: The Role of Social Support, Perceived Control, and Self-Blame," *Journal of Personality and Social Psychology* 48, no. 5 (May 1985); Ed Diener and Carol Diener, "Most People Are Happy," *Psychological Science* 7, no. 3 (May 1996); Roxanne Lee Silver, "Coping with an Undesirable Life Event: A Study of Early Reactions to Physical Disability" (Ph.D. diss., Northwestern University, 1982).

242 *For her dissertation:* H'Sien Hayward, "Posttraumatic Growth and Disability: On Happiness, Positivity, and Meaning" (Ph.D. diss., Harvard University, 2013).

243 *She conducted another study:* Ibid.

About the Author

JIM RENDON is a freelance journalist who writes about business, science, design, the environment, and many other topics. He's toured remote, ridgetop marijuana grows, gone cage diving with great white sharks, and visited maximum-security prisons and mental institutions in pursuit of a good story. His work has appeared in *The New York Times Magazine*, *The New York Times*, *Mother Jones*, *Marie Claire*, *Fortune*, *Outside*, and other publications. His previous book, *Super-Charged: How Hippies, Outlaws, and Scientists Reinvented Marijuana*, was published in 2012 by Timber Press.

He is a graduate of Ithaca College and the University of California, Berkeley Graduate School of Journalism. He is a former staff writer at *Metro*, Silicon Valley's alternative weekly, and *SmartMoney* magazine. He lives in Washington, D.C., with his wife and two children.